Urodynamics, Neurourology and Pelvic Floor Dysfunctions

Series Editor

Enrico Finazzi Agrò
Tor Vergata University
Urology Department
Rome, Italy

The aim of the book series is to highlight new knowledge on physiopathology, diagnosis and treatment in the fields of pelvic floor dysfunctions, incontinence and neurourology for specialists (urologists, gynecologists, neurologists, pediatricians, physiatrists), nurses, physiotherapists and institutions such as universities and hospitals.

More information about this series at http://www.springer.com/series/13503

Vincenzo Li Marzi · Maurizio Serati

Editors

Management of Pelvic Organ Prolapse

Current Controversies

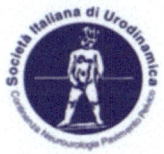

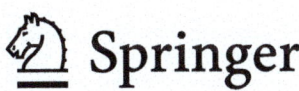

Editors
Vincenzo Li Marzi
Department of Urology
Careggi University Hospital
Florence, Italy

Maurizio Serati
Urogynecology Unit
University of Insubria
Varese, Italy

ISSN 2510-4047   ISSN 2510-4055   (electronic)
Urodynamics, Neurourology and Pelvic Floor Dysfunctions
ISBN 978-3-030-09642-7   ISBN 978-3-319-59195-7   (eBook)
https://doi.org/10.1007/978-3-319-59195-7

Printed on acid-free paper

This Springer imprint is published by the registered company Springer International Publishing AG part of Springer Nature
The registered company address is: Gewerbestrasse 11, 6330 Cham, Switzerland

Series Editor's Preface

It is my pleasure to introduce this volume entitled *Management of Pelvic Organ Prolapse*: *Current Controversies*, edited by Vincenzo Li Marzi and Maurizio Serati. The book is part of the series "Urodynamics, Neurourology and Pelvic Floor Dysfunctions," a series conceived by the Italian Society of Urodynamics (Società Italiana di UroDinamica—SIUD) to produce educational material for all the professionals involved in the management of urinary incontinence and lower urinary tract and pelvic floor dysfunctions.

As outlined by the editors, pelvic organ prolapse (POP) is certainly a frequent condition but, despite the large number of patients presenting this condition, several aspects of its evaluation and treatment are still controversial.

This book provides the most updated information on POP diagnosis and treatment and I am sure that many professionals, but in particular gynecologists and urologists, will find interesting data. SIUD hopes that this series in general and this book in particular may help to improve the quality of our diagnostic procedures and treatments and, ultimately, the patients' care.

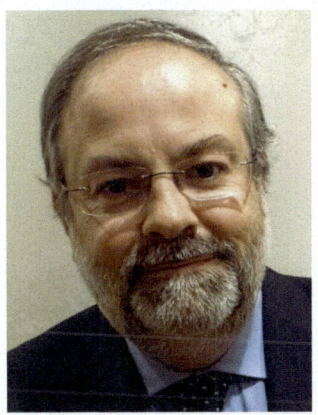

Prof. Enrico Finazzi Agrò
Associate Professor of Urology
Department of Experimental Medicine and Surgery
University of Rome Tor Vergata, Rome, Italy

President of the Italian Society of Urodynamics (SIUD), Florence, Italy

Preface

Pelvic organ prolapse (POP) is one of the most frequently reported and diagnosed uro-gynecological pathologies. Therefore, prolapse surgery is an increasingly important aspect of uro-gynecological practice.

During the last century, many efforts have been put by surgeons and researchers to investigate the pathophysiology, classification, and diagnosis of these disorders aiming to achieve effective treatment and improve quality of life.

Nonetheless, many aspects of POP assessment and treatment are still a matter of great debate, including the new findings about the role of genetic factors linked to POP incidence and the role of urodynamic evaluation.

Moreover, to date, there is still no "gold standard" for the treatment of vaginal prolapse.

This book provides a comprehensive overview of current hot topics in POP treatment, such as the use of prosthesis or native tissue reconstruction surgery as well as minimally invasive laparoscopic or robotic approaches. The role of hysterectomy for POP repair is also addressed.

Finally, an updated review of surgical outcomes after POP repair surgery, including perioperative complications, impact of surgery on bladder, sexual, and bowel function, and patient-reported quality of life outcomes, is outlined.

In 1966 TeLinde stated that "every honest surgeon of extensive and long experience will have to admit that he is not entirely and absolutely satisfied with his long term results of all his operations for prolapse and allied conditions." Nowadays, this scenario has not significantly changed. As such, we believe this book may be a reliable instrument for both urologists and gynecologists involved in the treatment of this challenging condition to improve patient care in routine clinical practice.

Florence, Italy   Vincenzo Li Marzi
Varese, Italy   Maurizio Serati

Contents

Contributors

Filippo Annino Department of Urology, San Donato Hospital, Arezzo, Italy

Daniele Bianchi Department of Experimental Medicine and Surgery, UOSD Functional Urology, Policlinico Tor Vergata, Rome, Italy

Antonella Biroli Neurologic and Autonomic Dysfunctions Rehabilitation Center, Physical Medicine and Rehabilitation Unit, San Giovanni Bosco Hospital, Torino, Italia

Andrea Braga Department of Obstetrics and Gynecology, EOC—Beata Vergine Hospital, Mendrisio, Switzerland

Rhiannon Bray Department of Obstetrics and Gynaecology, Imperial College NHS Trust, London, UK

Giorgio Caccia Department of Obstetrics and Gynecology, EOC—Beata Vergine Hospital, Mendrisio, Switzerland

Riccardo Campi Department of Urology, Careggi University Hospital, Florence, Italy

Elena Cattoni Department of Gynecology and Obstetrics, Regional Hospital of Lugano, Lugano, Switzerland

Elisabetta Costantini Department of Urology, University of Perugia, Perugia, Italy

Fabio Del Deo Department of Woman, Child and General and Specialistic Surgery, University of Campania Luigi Vanvitelli, Caserta, Italy

Giulio Del Popolo Department of Neuro-Urology, Careggi University Hospital, Florence, Italy

Alex Digesu Department of Obstetrics and Gynaecology, Imperial College NHS Trust, London, UK

Enrico Finazzi Agrò Department of Experimental Medicine and Surgery, UOSD Functional Urology, Policlinico Tor Vergata, Rome, Italy

Jacopo Frizzi Department of Urology, Careggi University Hospital, Florence, Italy

Richard Gaston Department of Urology, Clinique Saint Augustin, Bordeaux, France

Antonio Grimaldi Department of Woman, Child and General and Specialistic Surgery, University of Campania Luigi Vanvitelli, Caserta, Italy

Sharif I. M. F. Ismail Department of Obstetrics and Gynaecology, College of Medicine and Medical Sciences, Arabian Gulf University, Manama, Kingdom of Bahrain

Gian Franco Lamberti Department of Medicina Riabilitativa Ospedaliera di Fossano dell'ASL CN1, ASL CN1, Cuneo, Italy

Linda Leidi-Bulla Department of Gynecology and Obstetrics, Regional Hospital of Lugano, Lugano, Switzerland

Vincenzo Li Marzi Department of Urology, Careggi University Hospital, Florence, Italy

Michele Meschia Department of Obstetrics and Gynecology, "Fornaroli" Hospital, Magenta, Italy

Martina Milanesi Department of Urology, Careggi University Hospital, Florence, Italy

Andrea Minervini Department of Urology, Careggi University Hospital, Florence, Italy

Paulo Palma Department of Urology, Universidade de Estadual de Campinas, UNICAMP, São Paulo, Brazil

Diaa E. E. Rizk Department of Obstetrics and Gynaecology, College of Medicine and Medical Sciences, Arabian Gulf University, Manama, Kingdom of Bahrain

Maurizio Serati Department of Gynecology and Obstetrics, University of Insubria, Varese, Italy

Sergio Serni Department of Urology, Careggi University Hospital, Florence, Italy

Giampaolo Siena Department of Urology, Careggi University Hospital, Florence, Italy

Marco Soligo Urogynecology Unit, Obstetrics & Gynecology Department, Buzzi Hospital, University of Milan, Milan, Italy

Paola Sorice Department of Obstetrics and Gynecology, "Fornaroli" Hospital, Magenta, Italy

Marco Torella Department of Woman, Child and General and Specialistic Surgery, University of Campania Luigi Vanvitelli, Caserta, Italy

Gianni Vittori Department of Urology, Careggi University Hospital, Florence, Italy

Christian Wagner Department of Urology, Clinique Saint Augustin, Bordeaux, France

Part I

General Remarks

Surgical Anatomy for the Reconstructive Pelvic Surgeon

1

Paulo Palma and Elisabetta Costantini

1.1 Introduction

There are two important approaches to pelvic floor anatomy: functional anatomy and surgical anatomy.

The first has to do with the interaction between fascias, ligaments, nerves, and muscles in order to promote continence and support as the second deals with spaces and planes to restore pelvic floor defects.

1.2 Functional Anatomy of the Pelvic Floor

This part of anatomy is related to the functions of support of the pelvic organs as well as storage and elimination of feces and urine, continence, and incontinence. This is achieved basically by the dynamic interaction of the endopelvic fascia, pelvic floor muscles, perineal body, and perineal muscles [1, 2].

1.2.1 Pelvic Diaphragm

There are many controversies regarding the terminology of the levator ani muscle and related fascias. Accordingly, the pelvic diaphragm is made of the muscles levator ani and ischiococcygeus. The levator ani is made of three others:

P. Palma
Department of Urology, Universidade de Estadual de Campinas, UNICAMP,
São Paulo, Brazil

E. Costantini (✉)
Department of Surgical and Biomedical Science, Andrological and Urogynecological Clinic,
AOU Terni, University of Perugia, Perugia, Italy
e-mail: elisabetta.costantini@unipg.it

© Springer International Publishing AG, part of Springer Nature 2018
V. Li Marzi, M. Serati (eds.), *Management of Pelvic Organ Prolapse*,
Urodynamics, Neurourology and Pelvic Floor Dysfunctions,
https://doi.org/10.1007/978-3-319-59195-7_1

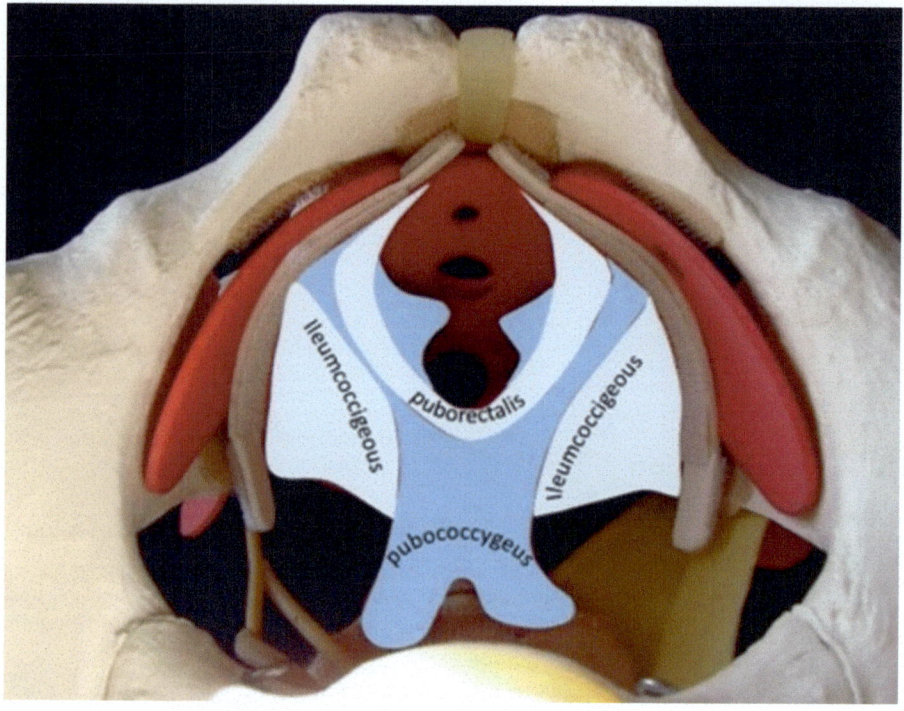

Fig. 1.1 Pubococcygeus muscle

1. Pubococcygeus (pubovisceral) muscle: Originates in the pubic bone and inserts in the coccyx (Fig. 1.1).
2. Puborectalis muscle: This muscle originates form the pubic bone and inserts in the contralateral side of the same bone, forming a sling that involves the distal rectum. Its contraction results in the rectoanal angle.
3. Iliococcygeus muscle: Originates at the arcus tendineus fascia pelvis, extends posteromedially, and inserts in the anterior aspect of the sacrum, resulting in the levator ani plateau.

Magnetic resonance studies, using tridimensional reconstruction, suggest a funnel appearance during the rest [3, 4].

The female perineum is rhomboidal in shape and delimited anteriorly by the pubic bone and symphysis, anterolaterally by the iliopubic ramus of the iliac bones, laterally by the ischial tuberosities, posterolaterally by the sacrotuberous ligaments, and posteriorly by the coccyx.

An imaginary line from one ischiatic tuberosity to the other divides the perineum in two triangles: urogenital (anterior) and anal (posteriorly) (Fig. 1.2) [4].

The muscles of the urogenital triangle are divided in superficial and deep, depending on the side of the perineal membrane (Fig. 1.3).

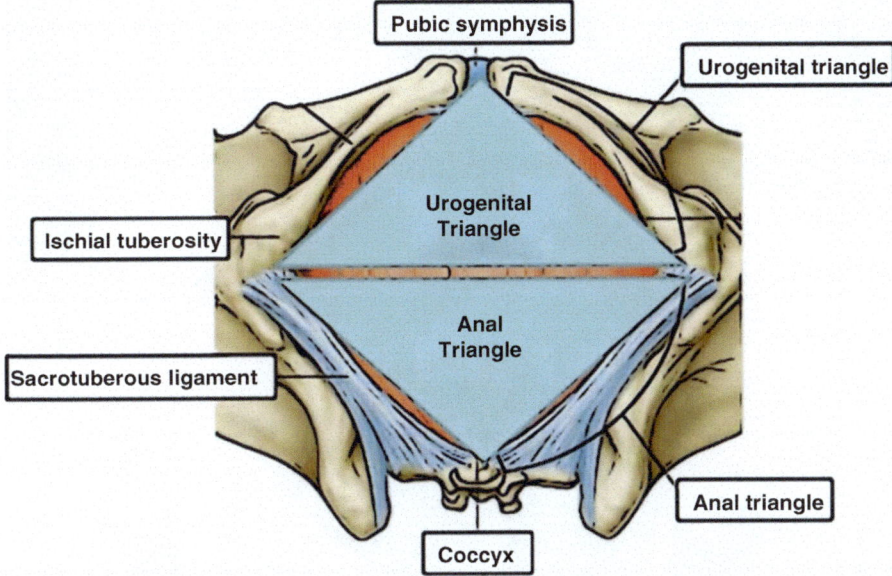

Fig. 1.2 Urogenital and anal triangles

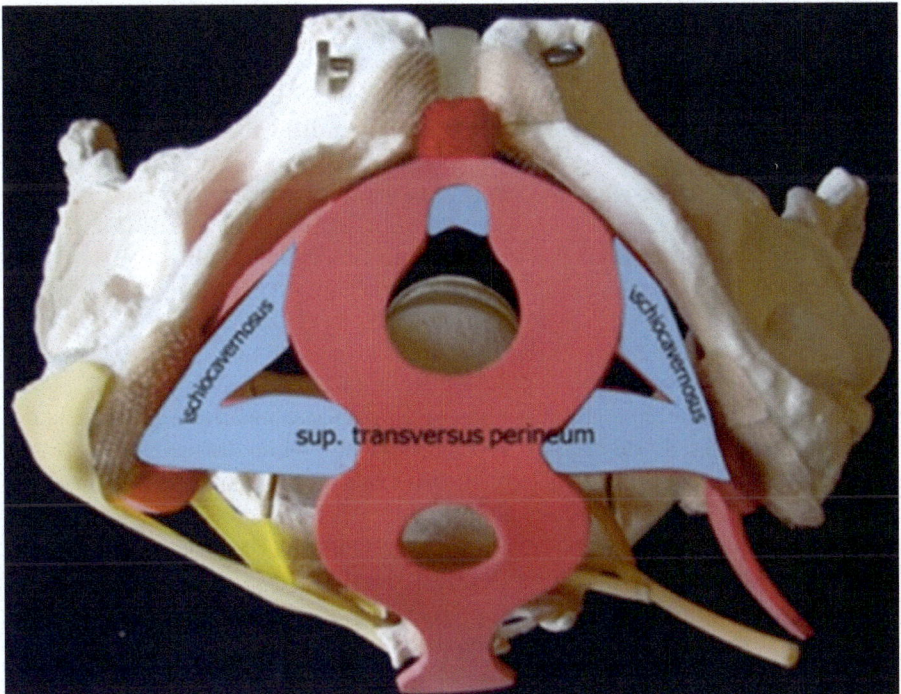

Fig. 1.3 Superficial muscles including bulbospongiosus muscles

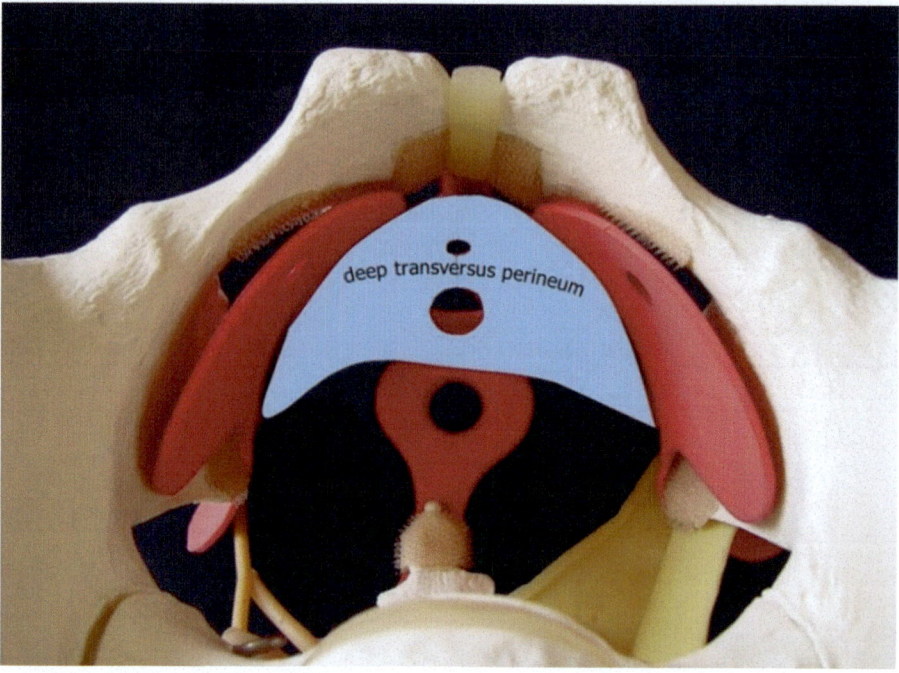

Fig. 1.4 Deep transversus perineum muscle

- Superficial transversus perineum: Originates at the ischiatic tuberosity and inserts at the perineal body.
- Bulbospongiosus: Originates at the perineal body and inserts at the corpus cavernosum of the clitoris.
- Ischiocavernosus: Originates at the ischial tuberosity and inserts at the crura of the clitoris.

On the other side, the deep muscles are (Fig. 1.4):

- Deep transversus perineum: Originates at the ischial tuberosity and inserts at the base of the perineal body.
- Urethrovaginal sphincter: Analogue to the bulbospongiosus muscle, surrounds the urethra and vaginal introitus.

1.2.1.1 Endopelvic Fascia
Refers to the fascia that connects viscera to the pelvic wall.

Didactically, the endopelvic fascia is named according to its localization and function [10–12].

Fig. 1.5 (*1*) Pericervical ring, (*2*) cardinal ligament, (*3*) sacrouterine ligament. Used with permission

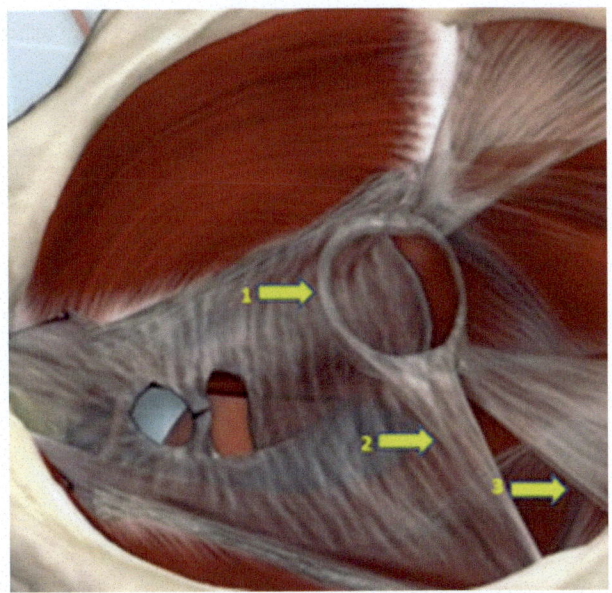

Cardinal-Sacrouterine Complex

This complex is made of the cardinal and sacrouterine ligaments and the paracolpos that forms a single structure that originates at the sacroiliac synostosis from S2 to S4 and inserts in the pericervical ring [3, 5]. This complex provides support to the uterus and the apex of the vagina (Fig. 1.5).

1.2.1.2 Pubocervical Fascia (Fig. 1.6)

1.2.1.3 Rectovaginal Fascia (Fig. 1.7)

1.2.1.4 Perineal Membrane and Perineal Body

The perineal membrane is a triangular-shaped structure (Fig. 1.8) on each side that inserts in the perineal body (Fig. 1.9). The lateral insertion includes ischiopubic ramus bone, ischiocavernosus muscles, and levator ani [6, 8].

This membrane stabilizes the perineal body and plays a role in the dynamics of the distal urethra.

The perineal body is a conic structure with the base looking at the perineum. At his point insert the external sphincter of the anus, the bulbocavernosus muscle, he transversus superficial and Deep of the perineum and its apex continues along with the rectovaginal fascia. This means that, indirectly, the perineal body is connected to the ischiopubic rami and ischiatic tuberosities by the perineal membrane and the transverse muscle of the perineum, to the coccyx by the external anal sphincter and anococcygeal ligament, and to the pelvic diaphragm by the rectovaginal fascia.

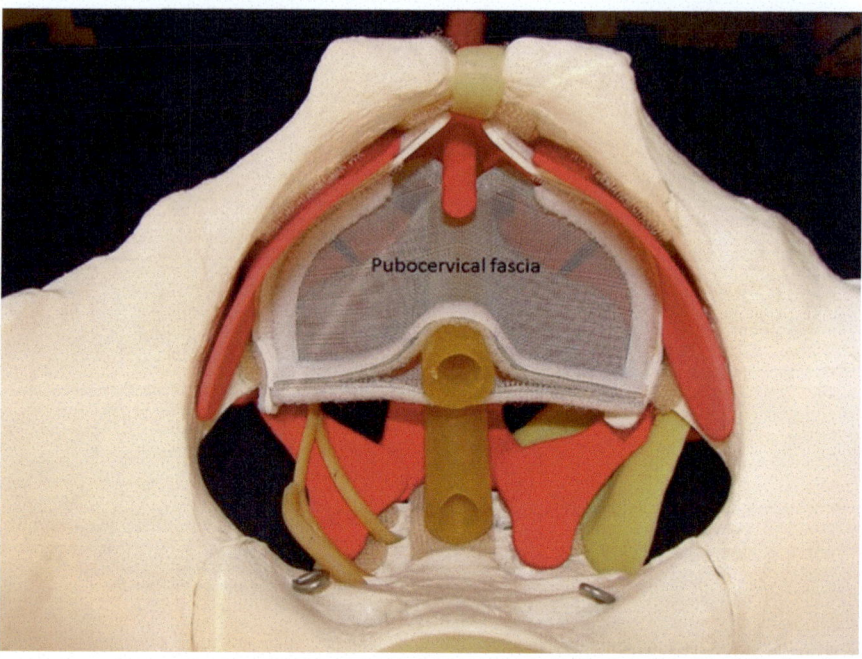

Fig. 1.6 The pubocervical fascia originates at the pubic bone and inserts laterally in the white line, arcus tendineus fascia pelvis, and proximally at the pericervical ring

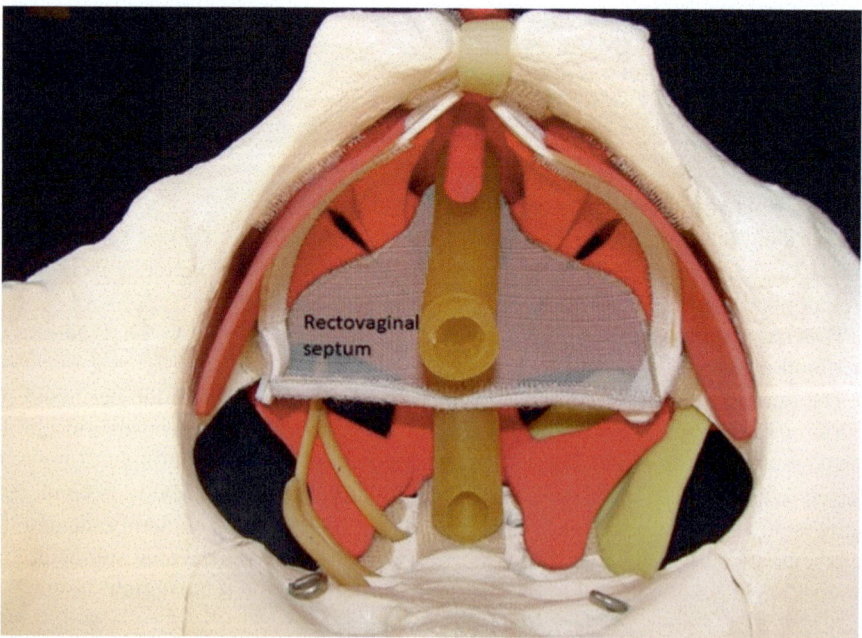

Fig. 1.7 The rectovaginal fascia is located between the rectum and the vagina and connects proximally to the cardinal uterosacral complex and levator ani plateau, laterally to the arcus tendineus of the rectovaginal fascia, and distally to the perineal body

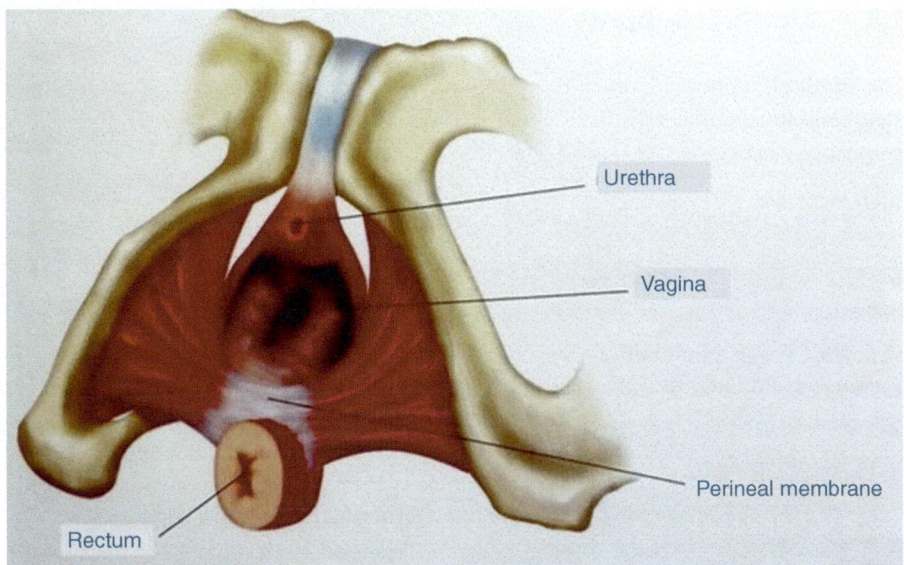

Fig. 1.8   Perineal membrane

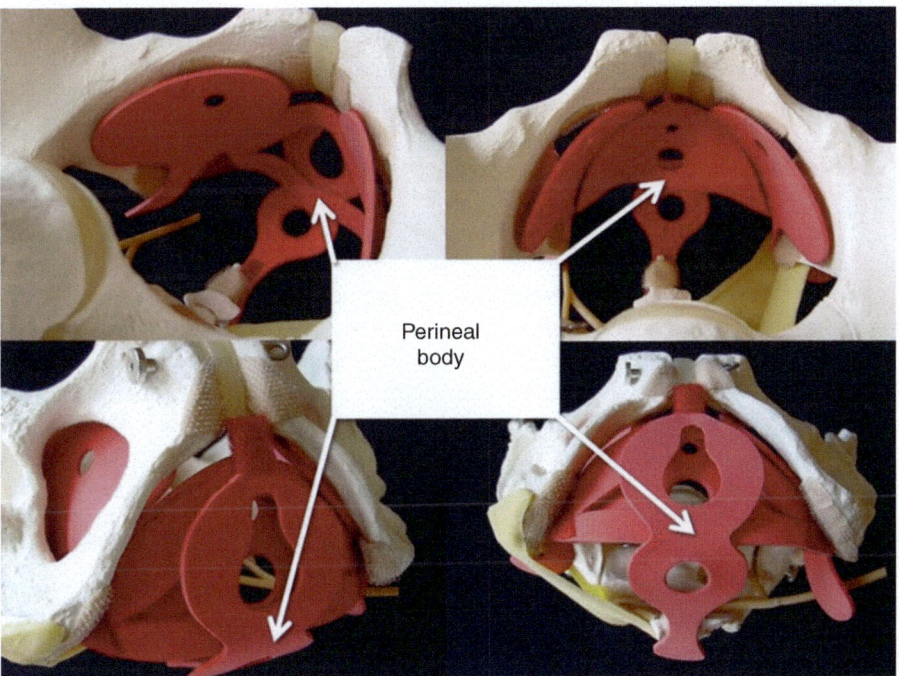

Fig. 1.9   Perineal body

1.3   Urethral Support

The urethral support involves the pubourethral ligaments, the urethropelvic ligament, and the vaginal wall itself (Figs. 1.10 and 1.11).

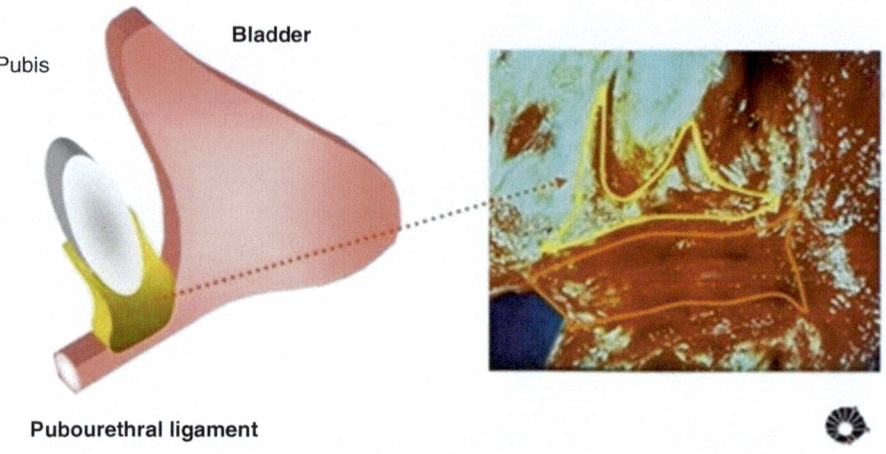

Fig. 1.10 The pubourethral ligament has a prepubic and a retropubic component

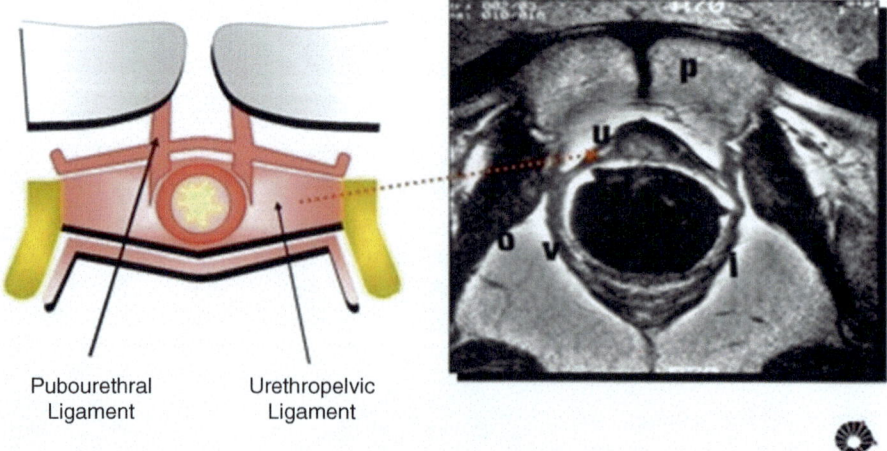

Fig. 1.11 The urethropelvic ligament is the only lateral fixation structure of the urethra

1.3.1   Level of Vaginal Support

The uterus and vagina are supported by the following structures, divided in three levels [5] (Fig. 1.12):

- Level I: Support of the uterus and upper third of the vagina by fibers of the complex cardinal-sacrouterine ligaments
- Level II: Lateral fixation of the vagina, provided by the pubocervical and rectovaginal fascia and its insertions in the arcus tendineus fascia pelvis and arcus tendineus fascia rectovaginalis, respectively
- Level III: Fusion of the vagina, pubovaginal muscle, and perineal body

1.3.1.1 Clinical Correlates

A tear at level I, that is, of the complex cardinal sacrouterine, may lead to uterine prolapse or vaginal vault prolapse.

On the other hand, a lesion of level II results in cystocele or rectocele.

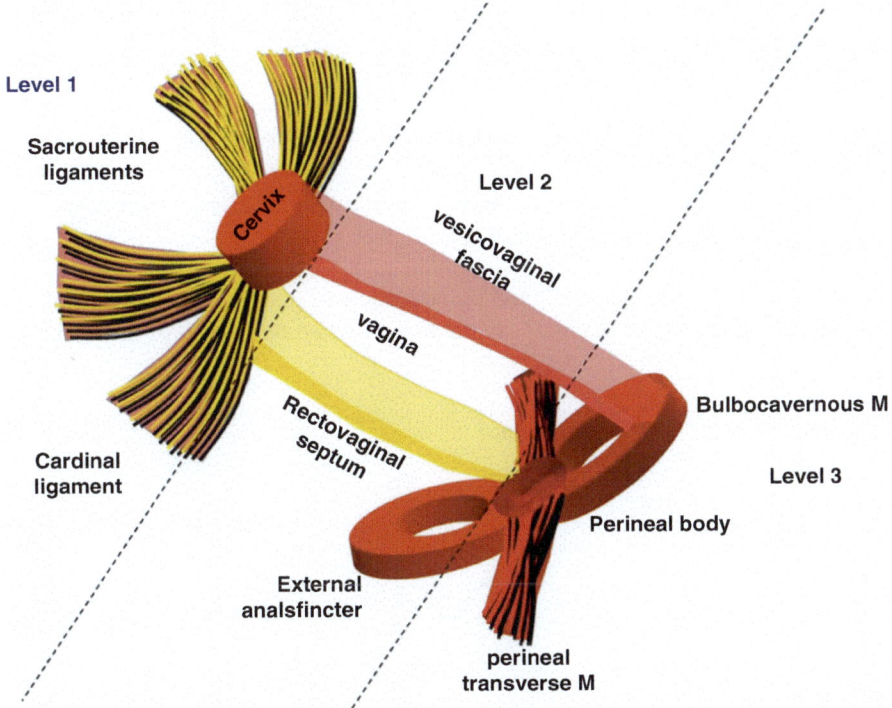

Fig. 1.12 Level of vaginal support

Finally, a lesion of level III that anteriorly supports elements of the urethra results in urethral hypermobility and posteriorly in laceration of the perineal body.

1.3.2   Mechanism of Urinary Continence and Micturition

The extrinsic mechanism of urinary continence is given mainly by two muscular groups [8]:

1. Anterior: Include the pubovaginal, ischiocavernosus, and pubococcygeal muscles.
2. Posterior: Iliococcygeus and ischiococcygeus muscles (levator plateau) and longitudinal anal muscle.

For continence, both muscular groups contract so that the proximal urethra is pulled posteriorly and the midurethra angulates, and it is coapted so that it is able to resist the increase in the abdominal pressure (Fig. 1.13).

During voiding, the relaxation of the anterior group along with the contraction of the posterior group results in funneling of the bladder neck and opening of the urethra allowing for normal voiding (Fig. 1.14).

1.3.3   Mechanism of Fecal Continence and Defecation

Anal continence and defecation occur in a similar way of urinary continence and voiding [9], that is, by two opposite forces:

1. Posterior group: Iliococcygeus and ischiococcygeus muscle contraction results in posterior tensioning of the rectovaginal fascia and posterior wall of the rectum.

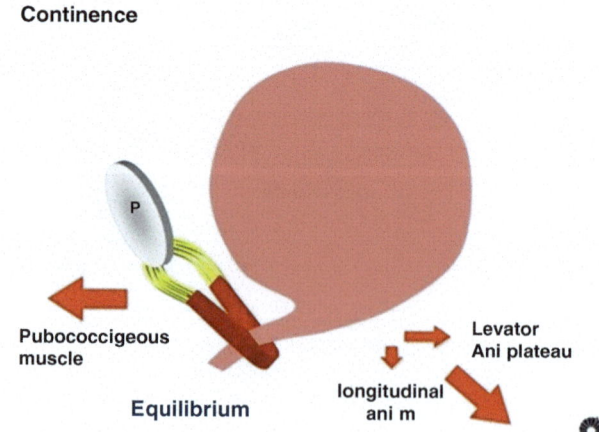

Fig. 1.13 Anterior and posterior forces in equilibrium

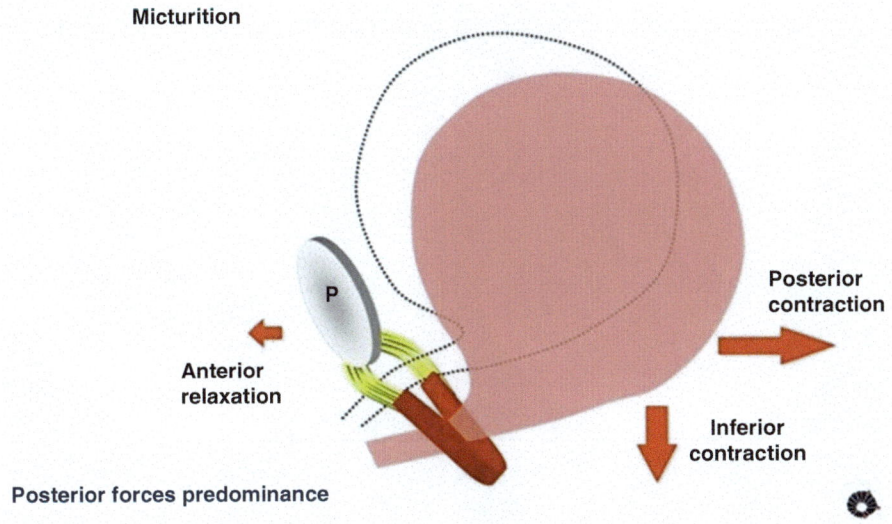

Micturition

Posterior contraction

Anterior relaxation

Inferior contraction

Posterior forces predominance

Fig. 1.14 During micturition, the posterior forces open the bladder neck and urethra

2. Anterior group: The puborectalis muscle contracts promoting the rectal angulation at the rectoanal transition.

For defecation, the levator plateau tension on the rectovaginal septum and posterior wall of the rectum and at the same time the puborectalis muscle relax. This synergistic action straights the anal canal. Finally, the internal and external sphincters relax the longitudinal muscle of the anus that contracts resulting in the opening of the anal canal.

For continence, the contraction of the levator plateau generates a posteroinferior vector, and the puborectalis contraction angulates the anal canal; at the same time, the contraction of the external anal sphincter moves the perineal body toward the anococcygeal ligament, promoting further angulation (Fig. 1.15).

1.3.4 Algorithm of Symptoms According to the Integral Theory

According to the Integral Theory [7], stress urinary incontinence and urgency may result from damaged ligaments and fascias, related to the urethra and vagina. Later on pelvic pain, voiding, and anal symptoms were added.

The systematization of these symptoms is shown in Table 1.1.

It is important to underline that these compartments are different from the levels of support proposed by DeLancey [5]. The anterior compartment includes the puborethral and urethropelvic ligaments, both level III according to DeLancey [5].

The median compartment is composed of the pubocervical fascia and its insertions (level II), and the posterior compartment includes the complex cardinal sacrouterine ligaments, rectovaginal fascia, and perineal body, respectively, levels I, II, and III according to DeLancey.

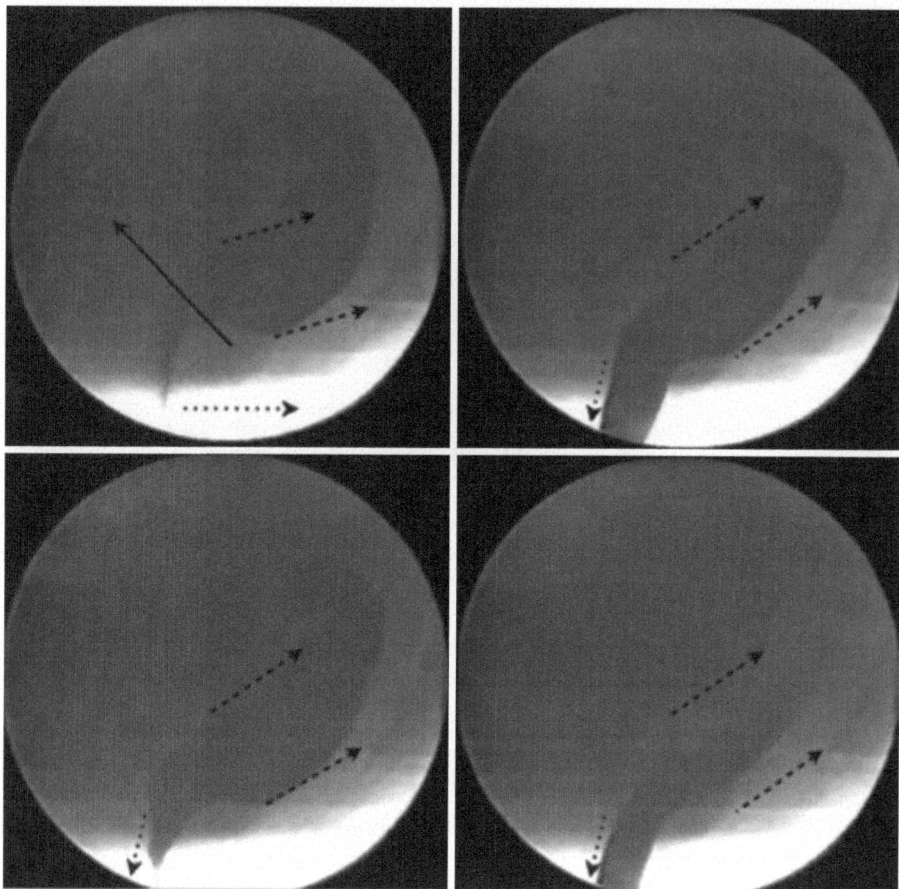

Fig. 1.15 Anal continence and defecation

1.3.4.1 Symptoms from the Anterior Compartment

The anterior compartment defects produce stress urinary incontinence, urgency, and anal incontinence.

Urinary incontinence is easy to understand since damage to the elements of support of the urethra impairs the proper coaptation of the urethral lumen.

The urgency is derived from the urethral afferent nerves stimulation, since inadequate coaptation allows for the presence of urine in the proximal urethra, and this is interpreted as maximum bladder capacity, even with small volume in the bladder.

More difficult is to correlate anal incontinence, but remember that the urethral support ligaments help to support the insertion of the puborectalis muscle. In order to be effective, the muscular contraction needs good contra-traction at its insertion. Therefore, lesion of the urethral ligaments may impair the tonus of the puborectalis muscle, diminishing the anorectal angulation and may lead to anal incontinence.

Table 1.1 Algorithm of symptoms

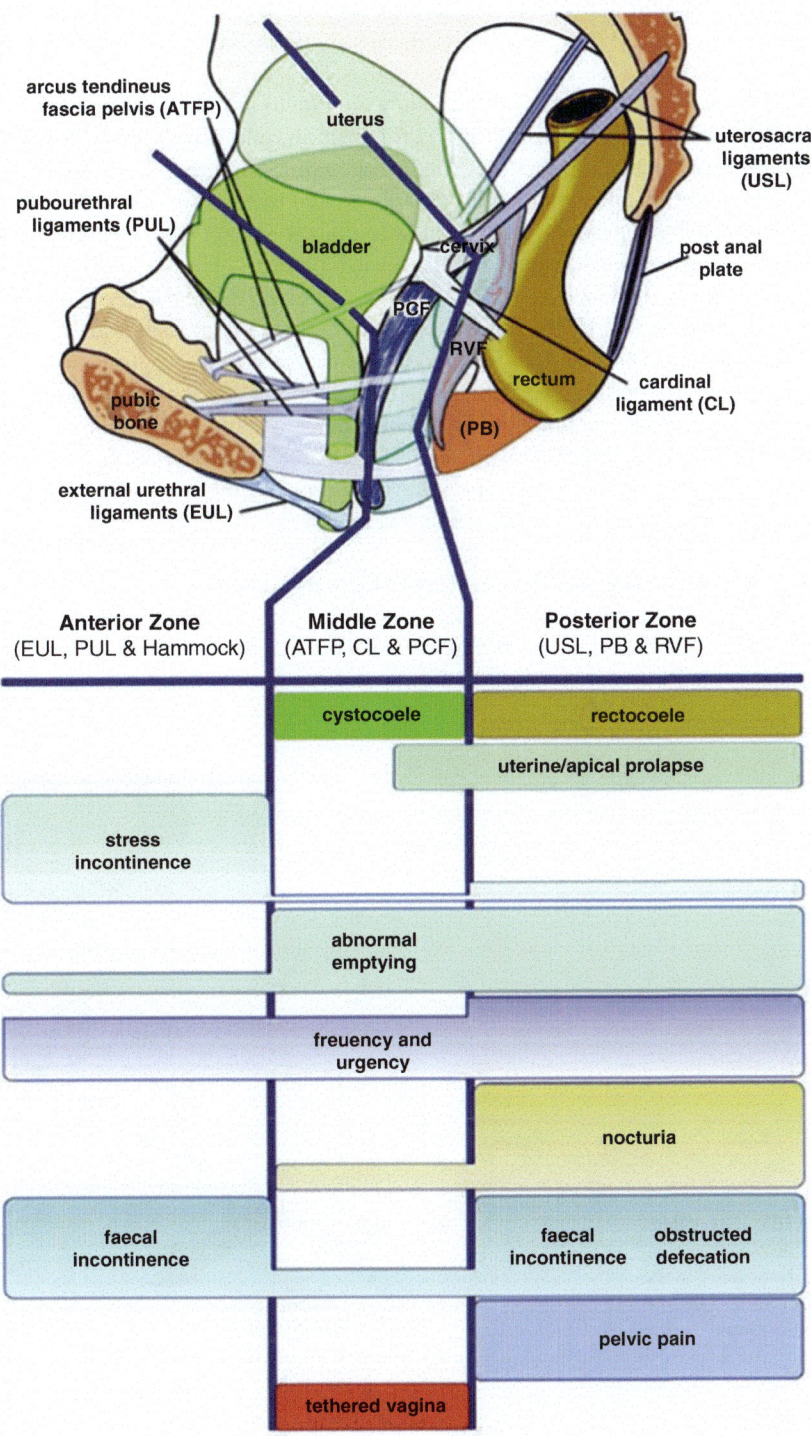

1.3.4.2 Symptoms from the Middle Compartment

The middle compartment refers to the pubocervical fascia and its insertion at the ATFP and pericervical ring. Damage to these structures may cause urgency, voiding dysfunction, nocturia, and pelvic pain.

The symptoms of urgency and frequency are due to overstimulation of the afferents of the bladder. The inhibition of the micturition reflex depends on the simultaneous and coordinated contraction of the striated musculature of the pelvic floor so that the mid-urethra and proximal urethra are closed by traction of the urethral ligaments and also by suppressing the stimulation of the stretch receptor in the trigone (Fig. 1.16). Due to the contraction of the levator plateau.

When a tear in the fascia is present or even a damage to the pericervical ring, the force transmission will be inadequate, and the hydrostatic pressure due to the column of urine will continue to be exerted on the receptor in the trigone.

The brain will interpret this signal as a full bladder, even at small volumes.

Voiding symptoms such as low flow, hesitancy, dribbling, and incomplete voiding are due to the impaired transmission of the force generated by the levator plateau to the trigone. As described previously, the posterior force is needed for the urethral opening during the voiding phase (Fig. 1.17).

1.3.4.3 Symptoms from the Posterior Compartment

In the posterior compartment are located the complex cardinal sacrouterine ligaments, rectovaginal fascia, and perineal body (Fig. 1.18) so that this compartment correlates with all symptoms derived from pelvic support damage to some extent.

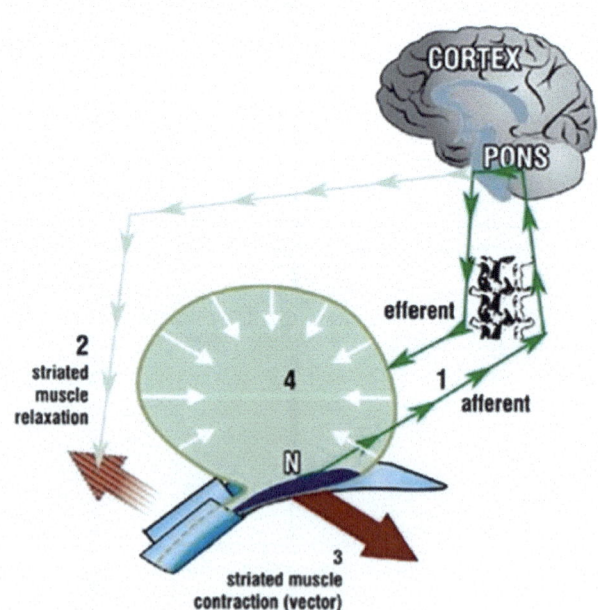

Fig. 1.16 Micturition reflex. Notice the integration between the pelvic floor and the nervous system

Fig. 1.17 Posterior and inferior forces allow for the opening of the bladder neck and urethra

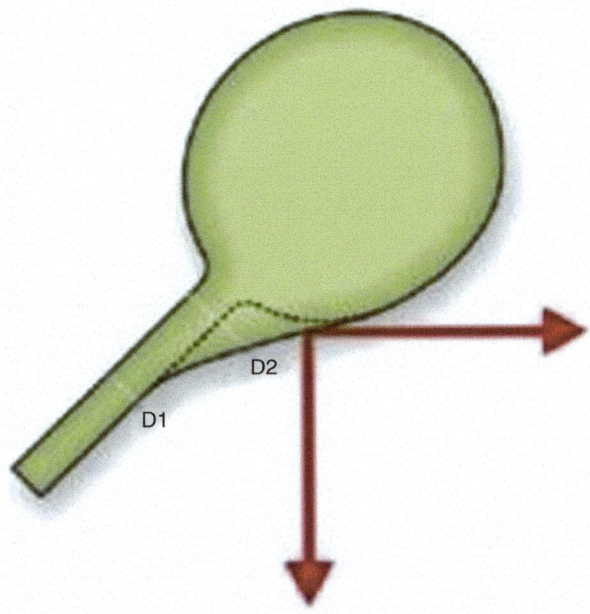

Fig. 1.18 Components of the posterior compartment

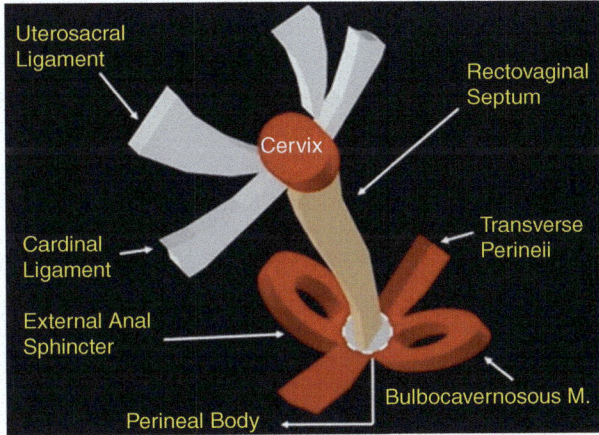

- Urgency: May be due to lesion of the cardinal sacrouterine complex that prevents the tension due to the contraction of the levator plateau to be transmitted to the pericervical ring and rectovaginal fascia (Fig. 1.19).
- Nocturia: Related to incomplete voiding and urine residuals.
- Pelvic pain: The nerve fibers that travel along the sacrouterine cardinal complex are distended by the gravity (G), producing pelvic pain.

Fig. 1.19 Defect in the
sacrouterine ligaments
impairs bladder neck and
urethra opening and
bladder base support
(urgency)

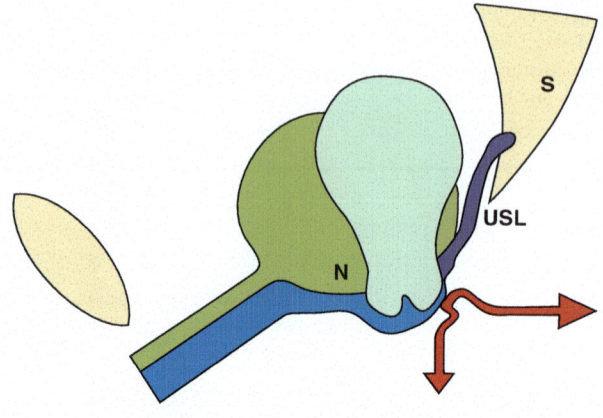

Conclusion

Pelvic floor dysfunction and symptoms may have the same etiopathology. There is clinical correlation between the pelvic floor muscle and components of the endopelvic fascia, and therefore symptoms are generally associated.

It is important to know these correlations in order to deliver better care to the patients.

References

1. DeLancey JO. Structural aspects of the extrinsic continence mechanism. Obstet Gynecol. 1988;72(3 Pt 1):296–301.
2. Kearney R, Sawhney R, DeLancey JO. Levator ani muscle anatomy evaluated by origin—insertion pairs. Obstet Gynecol. 2004;104(1):168–73.
3. DeLancey JO. Surgical anatomy fo the female pelvic floor. In: TeLinde's operative gynecology. 9th ed. Baltimore: Lippincot Williams & Wilkins; 2003.
4. Barber M. Contemporary views on female pelvic anatomy. Cleveland Clin J Med. 2005;72(Suppl. 4):S3–11.
5. DeLancey JO. Anatomic aspects of vaginal eversion after hysterectomy. Am J Obstet Gynecol. 1992;166:1717–28.
6. DeLancey JO. Structural anatomy of the posterior pelvic compartment as it relates torectocele. Am J Obstet Gynecol. 1999;180(4):815–23.
7. Stein TA, DeLancey JO. Structure of the perineal membrane in females: gross and microscopic anatomy. Obstet Gynecol. 2008;111(3):686–93. 8.
8. Petros PE, Ulmsten UI. An integral theory and its method for the diagnosis and management of female urinary incontinence. Scand J Urol Nephrol Suppl. 1993;153:1–93.
9. Petros PE, Swash M. The musculo-elastic theory of anorectal function and dysfunction. Pelviperineology. 2008;27:89–93. Disponível em: www.pelviperineology.org.
10. Petros PE, Ulmsten U. An integral theory of female urinary incontinence. Acta Obstet Gynecol Scand. 1990;69(Suppl 153):1–79.
11. Petros PE, Ulmsten UI. Bladder instability in women: a premature activation of the micturition reflex. Neurourol Urod. 1993;12:235–9.
12. Palma P, Riccetto C, Fraga R, Portugal S, Dambros M, Rincón ME, Silveira A, Netto NR Jr. Anatomia tridimensional y cirugia virtual para procedimientos transobturatrizes. Actas Urol Esp. 2007;31(4):361–5.

Pelvic Organ Prolapse: Pathophysiology and Epidemiology

2

Andrea Braga and Giorgio Caccia

The pelvic floor is the bottom of the pelvic cavity. It consists of several components: peritoneum, pelvic viscera, endopelvic fascia, levator ani muscles, perineal membrane, and superficial genital muscles. The support for all these structures comes from connections to the bony pelvis and its attached muscles. Furthermore, viscera play an important role in forming the pelvic floor through their connections with structures, such as the cardinal and uterosacral ligaments [1]. For these reasons, it should not be considered as a single compartment but as a complex of structures in strong synergism, to ensure multiple functions. The interaction and integrity of muscular, connective, and nerve structures is essential to guarantee normal pelvic organ support. If one of these factors fails, the other might be able to compensate to a certain degree until pelvic organ prolapse occurs [2]. The International Urogynecological Association (IUGA) and International Continence Society (ICS), in their joint report, defined the prolapse as the descent of one or more of the anterior vaginal wall, posterior vaginal wall, the uterus (cervix), or the apex of the vagina (vaginal vault or cuff scar after hysterectomy). The presence of any such sign should be correlated with relevant POP symptoms. More commonly, this correlation would occur at the level of the hymen or beyond. Prolapse symptoms are vaginal bulging, pelvic pressure, bleeding, discharge, infection, splinting/digitation, and low back pain. These are generally worse at the times when gravity might make the prolapse worse (e.g. after long periods of standing or exercise) and better when gravity is not a factor, for example, lying supine.

Historically, the severity of prolapse was graded using several classification systems that were not easily reproduced or communicated in a standard way among clinicians [2]. The pelvic organ prolapse quantification (POPQ) system, introduced

A. Braga (✉) · G. Caccia
Department of Obstetrics and Gynecology, EOC—Beata Vergine Hospital,
Mendrisio, Switzerland
e-mail: andrea.braga@eoc.ch; giorgio.caccia@eoc.ch

© Springer International Publishing AG, part of Springer Nature 2018
V. Li Marzi, M. Serati (eds.), *Management of Pelvic Organ Prolapse*,
Urodynamics, Neurourology and Pelvic Floor Dysfunctions,
https://doi.org/10.1007/978-3-319-59195-7_2

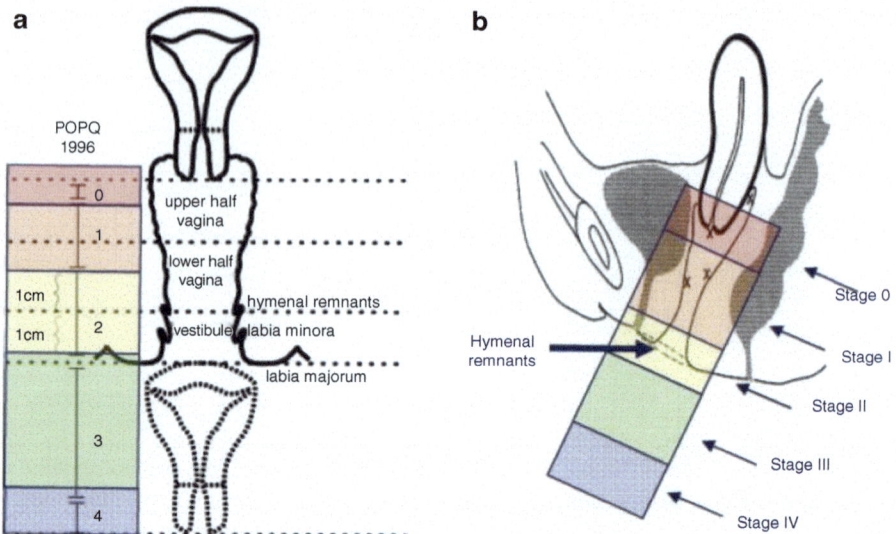

Fig. 2.1 (**a**, **b**) Prolapse staging—0, 1, 2, 3, and 4 (From IUGA/ICS Joint Report on the Terminology for Female Pelvic Floor Dysfunction, 2010 [3])

in 1996, has become the standard classification system [3]. It defines prolapse by measuring the descent of specific segments of the reproductive tract during Valsalva strain relative to a fixed point, the hymen (Fig. 2.1a, b).

It has proven interobserver and intraobserver reliability [4] and is the system used most commonly in the medical literature [5, 6]. However, it can be difficult to apply clinically without practice, repetition, and continuous use. A simplified POPQ system was developed by IUGA to provide a less cumbersome exam tool and to ensure its use in routine clinical practice [7]. Although these systems provide a topographic map of the vagina, it does not consider symptoms and bothers perceived by the woman. Determining POP based on self-reported symptoms is difficult because of the lack of specificity and sensitivity of most symptoms attributed to pelvic organ prolapse and the fact that prolapse above the level of the hymeneal ring is usually asymptomatic. The only exception appears to be a sensation of bulging into the vagina, which is most strongly associated with prolapse at or below the hymeneal ring [8]. The hymen seems to be an important "cut-off point" for symptom development. As a matter of fact, a recent study demonstrated that the feeling of something bulging in or dropping out of their vagina had a sensitivity of 84% and a specificity of 94% for POP.

2.1 Prevalence and Incidence of POP

In the United States, pelvic organ prolapse (POP) is the cause of more than 300,000 surgical procedures per year (22.7 per 10,000 women) with 13–25% leading to reoperation, with an estimated burden to the healthcare system of $1 billion. It is clear that the treatment of genital prolapse is not only important for women's health and quality of life, but it also has a strong impact on the planning and management of women's health services [9].

It's difficult to estimate the real prevalence of prolapse. The reason is that exist different classification systems used for diagnosis, several studies reported different prolapse rates depending on symptomatic or asymptomatic condition, and it is unknown how many women do not seek medical care. Indeed, POP is an underreported condition and occurs in up to 50% of parous women, but only 10–20% of those seek evaluation for their condition [10]. The overall prevalence of POP varies significantly depending upon the definition used, ranging from 3 to 50% (Table 2.1). When based on symptoms, it is 3–6%; when based on examination, it is 41–50%, because mild prolapse on examination is common and frequently asymptomatic [11]. Distinguishing symptomatic and asymptomatic POP is clinically relevant for its treatment. Nevertheless there are few high-quality data regarding the prevalence of symptomatic POP. Nygaard et al. [12], in a cross-sectional study, on 1961 women aged 20–80 years, defined symptomatic prolapse as a positive response to the question derived from the Pelvic Floor Distress Inventory [13], "Do you experience bulging or something falling out you can see or feel in the vaginal area?" and

Table 2.1 Prevalence and incidence of pelvic organ prolapse (POP)

Study	Definition	Prevalence	Incidence	Country
Rortveit [22]	Symptom-based	5.7%		The United States
Nygaard [12]	Symptom-based	2.9%		The United States
Hendrix [14]	WHI study, Examination	Any prolapse: 41.1% Cystocele: 34.3% Rectocele: 18.6% Uterine: 14.2%		The United States
Swift [15]	Examination	6.4% stage 0 43.3% stage 1 47.7% stage 2 2.6% stage 3		The United States
Handa [23]	WHI study, Examination	Cystocele: 24.6% Rectocele: 12.9% Uterine: 3.8%	Cystocele: 0.3/100 Rectocele: 5.7/100 Uterine: 1.5/100	The United States
Nygaard [24]	Examination	2.3% stage 0 33% stage 1 63% stage 2 1.9% stage 3		The United States
Bradley [18]	Examination	23.5–49.9%	26%/1 year 40%/3 year	The United States
Marchionni [25]	Examination	Vault prolapse: 12%		Italy
Aigmueller [26]	Examination	Vault prolapse: 6–8%		Austria

Adapted from Maher et al. [11]

reported a 2.9% prevalence of symptomatic POP. A positive response was correlated with the presence of a vaginal bulge on examination. However, prolapse
assessment using only questionnaires underreports the true prevalence of prolapse
based on clinical examination as surveys are likely to only identify women with
advanced prolapse. Rates of asymptomatic POP are probably even higher. In a
cross-sectional analysis of 16,616 women, who enrolled in the Women's Health
Initiative Hormone Replacement Therapy Clinical Trial, the rate of prolapse, evaluated with non-validated physical examination, was 41% in women with uterus (with
34.3% having cystocele, 14.2% having uterine prolapse, and 18.6% having rectocele) and 38% in women without a uterus (with 32.9% having cystocele and 18.3%
having rectocele) [14]. Swift et al., in an observational study performed on 497
women aged 18–82 years old, who were seen in an outpatient clinic for routine
gynaecologic care and were assessed using the POPQ system, reported that 6.4% of
patients had POPQ stage 0, 43.3% had stage 1, 47.7% had stage 2, and 2.6% had
stage 3. No subjects examined had POPQ system stage 4 prolapse [15]. These data
demonstrate that most women have some degree of POP. Nevertheless, there is a
lack of studies correlating degree of prolapse on physical exam to symptomatic
bother. For these reasons, in order to establish true prevalence rates and to follow the
natural history and progression of POP in the general population in the future, a
large-scale observational study including premenopausal and postmenopausal
women would need to be performed [16].

About incidence and natural history of POP, there is poor knowledge. On examination anterior compartment prolapse is the most frequently reported site of prolapse and is detected twice as often as posterior compartment defects and three
times more commonly than apical prolapse. Following hysterectomy 6–12% of
women will develop vaginal vault prolapse, and in two thirds of these cases, multi-
compartment prolapse is present [11]. The reported incidence for cystocele is
around 9 per 100 women-years, 6 per 100 women-years for rectocele, and 1.5 per
100 women-years for uterine prolapse [17]. Bradley et al. reported an overall
1-year and 3-year prolapse incidence of 26% and 40%, respectively, while regression rates were 21% and 19%, respectively [18]. Older parous women are more
likely to develop new or progressive POP than to show regression. The peak incidence of prolapse symptoms is between ages of 70 and 79, while POP symptoms
are still relatively common in younger women (Fig. 2.2) [19]. The annual incidence of POP surgery is stated to be between 1.5 and 1.8 cases per 1000 women-
years, with the incidence peaking in women between 60 and 69 years. Surprisingly,
high numbers of younger women were also undergoing surgical treatment, reflect-
ing a similarity in the prolapse symptoms reported in younger women by Luber
et al. [19, 20].

Given that advancing age is a major risk factor for the development of POP, there
will be an increasing number of female patients presenting to healthcare providers
with POP. In fact, Wu et al. [21] have predicted, on the basis of population growth
statistics in the United States, that by 2050 the number of women suffering from
symptomatic POP will increase by a minimum of 46%, from 3.3 up to 4.9 million
women and in a "worst-case scenario" up to 200% or 9.2 million women with POP.

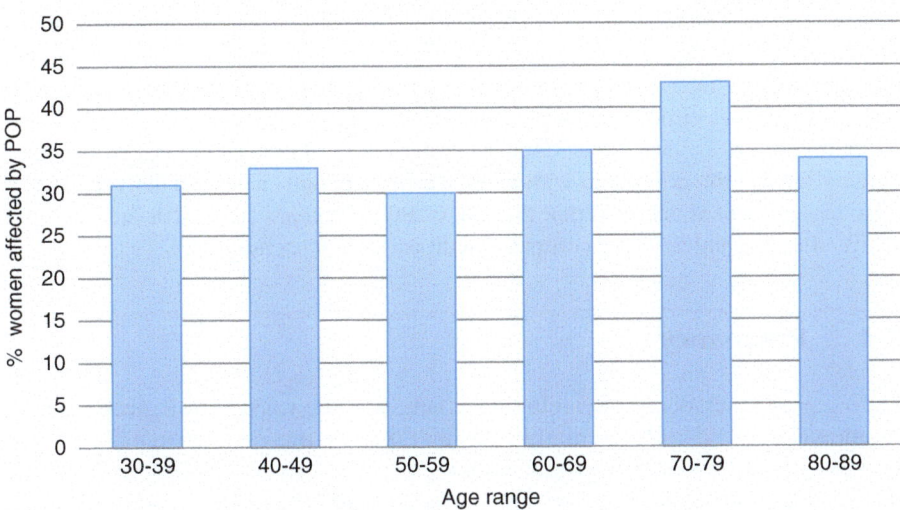

Fig. 2.2 Distribution of POP among women seeking care, USA, 2000 (modified from Barber et al. [11])

2.2   Pathophysiology of POP

The aetiology of pelvic organ prolapse is multifactorial with contributions from both environmental and genetic risk factors.

2.3   Childbirth

It is widely accepted that childbirth is a significant risk factor for pelvic organ prolapse, presumably due to overt or occult pelvic floor tissue trauma. This increased risk is thought to occur secondary to stretching, compression, or avulsion during labour that causes structural compromise and/or denervation to the levator ani musculature (LAM), which is associated with pelvic organ prolapse. The occurrence of levator trauma postpartum is reported to be between 15 and 39.5% with ultrasound [27] and between 17.7 and 19.1% with MRI [28]. Dietz et al. showed that avulsion of the inferomedial aspects of the LAM from the pelvic side-wall occurred in approximately one third of all women delivered vaginally and suggests that older age at first delivery is a risk factor for such trauma [29]. These women have about twice as likely to show pelvic organ prolapse of stage 2 or higher than those without LAM, with an increased risk of cystocele and uterine prolapse [30]. In the prospective Oxford Family Planning Association study [31], childbirth was the single strongest risk factor for developing prolapse in women under 59 years of age and the risk increased by every delivery. In fact compared with nulliparous women, women with 1 child were 4 times more likely and women with 2 children were 8.4 times more likely to experience POP that required hospital admission. This indicates that among parous women, 75% of prolapse can be attributed to pregnancy and childbirth [32]. Caesarean section seems to protect against prolapse development. Leijonhufvud et al. demonstrated that women who had only vaginal childbirths were associated with a significantly increased risk (hazard ratio, 9.2; 95% confidence interval, 7.0–12.1) of pelvic organ prolapse surgery later in life compared with women who only had caesarean deliveries [33]. Also Gyhagen et al. showed that the risk of POP 20 years after birth increased by 255% after vaginal delivery compared with caesarean section [34].

2.4 Pregnancy

During pregnancy occur physiological changes in the vaginal wall, secondary to hormonal-induced collagen alterations, that include increased distensibility and decreased stiffness and maximal stress [35]. The effect of pregnancy on the development of pelvic organ prolapse was evaluated by O'Boyle et al. [36] in a series of 135 nulliparous pregnant women. POPQ stage assignments and POPQ component measurements were compared for first-, second-, and third-trimester examinations. Overall POPQ stage was significantly higher in the third trimester than in the first. These findings probably represent normal physiological changes of the pelvic floor during pregnancy but suggest that significant changes may be objectively demonstrated prior to delivery. The same author in a case-control study compared 21 nulliparous nonpregnant women with 21 nulliparous pregnant women and found that all patients in the nonpregnant group had a POPQ stage of 0 or 1, whereas 47.6% of the pregnant subjects had POPQ stage 2 ($p < 0.001$). Overall POPQ stage was higher in the third trimester than in the first ($p = 0.001$) [37]. Also, Sze et al. reported that 46% of 94 nulliparous women had pelvic organ prolapse at their 36-week antepartum visit. Of them, 26% had a stage 2 prolapse [38].

2.5 Obstetric Factors

Other obstetric factors in addition to parity and pregnancy can influence the risk of prolapse. Operative vaginal delivery with the use of forceps has been associated with three times the odds of levator trauma [39] and may increase the odds of levator injury and resultant prolapse. Handa et al. [40] found that operative vaginal birth significantly increased the risk for all pelvic floor disorders, especially pelvic organ prolapse (OR 7.5, 95% CI 2.7–20.9). In contrast, Uma et al. [41] found no significant association between pelvic organ prolapse and forceps delivery (OR 0.9, 95% CI 0.7–1.2).

Although less consistently, also infant birth weight (>4500 g), vaginal delivery of a macrosomic infant, prolonged second stage of labour, and age < 25 years at first delivery were associated with development of POP [42, 43].

2.6   Obesity

Elevated body mass index >25 is associated with a twofold higher risk of having prolapse when compared with normal weight [44]. Increased waist circumference was associated with more pelvic organ prolapse in some studies, especially for progressive rectocele [23, 24]. Handa et al. demonstrated this for cystocele [23]. While weight gain is a risk factor for developing prolapse, weight loss does not appear to be significantly associated with regression of POP, suggesting that damage to the pelvic floor related to weight gain might be irreversible [45]. However, obese women, after surgically induced weight loss, showed an improvement in anterior vaginal support and pelvic floor symptoms [46].

2.7   Age

There are wide evidences that POP increases with advancing age. Swift et al., in a cross-sectional study of 1004 women (aged 18–83 years) who attended their annual gynaecological examination, demonstrated that the prevalence of this disorder rose by about 40% with every decade of life [44]. The annual incidence of POP surgery is stated to be between 1.5 and 1.8 cases per 1000 women-years, with the incidence peaking in women between 60 and 69 years [47, 48]. Shah et al. [48] also demonstrated a peak incidence in 70-year-old women (Fig. 2.3). In the NHANES study described above, the proportion of women with symptomatic prolapse was lowest in young women and then remained fairly constant over age 40 years: ages 20 to 39 (1.6%), 40 to 59 (3.8%), 60 to 79 (3.0%), and ≥80 (4.1%) [12]. In the Women's

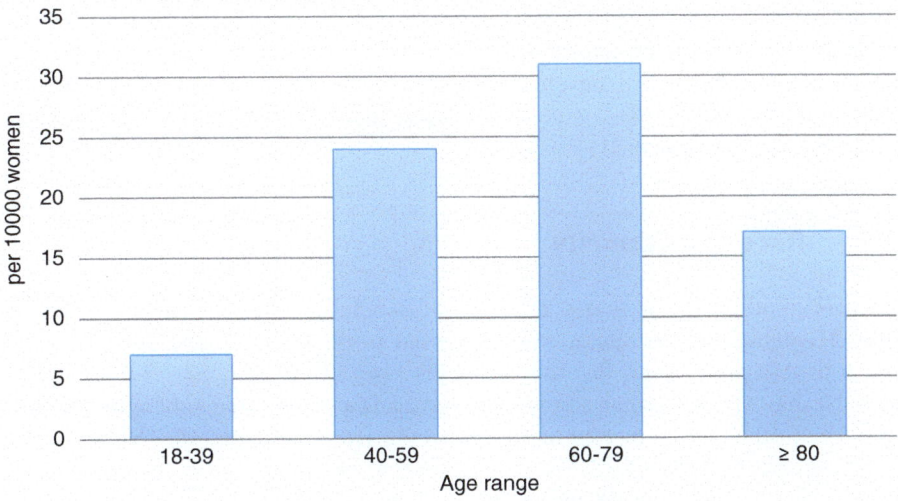

Fig. 2.3 Surgical treatment for POP/rate per 10,000 women (modified from Barber et al. [11])

Health Initiative, American women aged 60–69 years (OR1.2; 95% CI: 1.0–1.3) and 70–79 years (OR 1.4; 95%CI: 1.2–1.6) had a higher risk of prolapse than did those aged 50–59 [14].

2.8   Inheritance and Genetic Factors

Recently, a large body of evidence regarding familial transmission of pelvic organ prolapse has been shown. Uncontrolled studies reported disparate estimates of the proportion of prolapse patients with a family history of prolapse. First-degree family history of prolapse seems to increase the risk of prolapse as carried out by Chiaffarino et al. [49]. In fact their data showed that the risk of urogenital prolapse was higher in women with mother or sisters reporting the condition (the ORs were, respectively, 3.2 (95% CI 1.1–7.6) and 2.4 (95% CI 1.0–5.6)) in comparison with women whose mother or sisters reported no prolapse. Jack et al. [50], in their study on familial transmission of genitovaginal prolapse, identified 10 patients with stage 3 and 4 prolapse, younger than 55 years (average age 37), a family history of prolapse, with a mean number of deliveries of 1.8, and with a mean birth weight of 8 lbs. Genetic analysis of the inheritance pattern within these families demonstrated that pelvic organ prolapse segregated in a dominant fashion with incomplete penetrance in these families. The authors demonstrated that the relative risk of POP among siblings of young women affected of POP was five times higher than the general population. In the larger Swedish twin registry of 3376 monozygotic and 5067 dizygotic female twin pairs, a greater twin similarity among the monozygotic twins was found, indicating the influence of a genetic component to the aetiology of pelvic organ prolapse. Genetic and non-shared environmental factors seemed to contribute equally to the development of pelvic floor disorders in these women, about 40% for each factor [51]. High concordance of pelvic organ prolapse in nulliparous and parous sister pairs was found by Buchsbaum et al., suggesting a familial predisposition toward developing this condition [52]. Furthermore, genetic variants present in families with an increased incidence of pelvic organ prolapse [52] have been documented [53–56].

2.9   Race and Ethnicity

Race is another factor that seems to be associated with the development of POP. Hispanic and European women appear to be at higher risk for POP than those of African, Asian, or other descents [14, 22, 44, 57, 58]. Some studies suggest that African-American women have a lower prevalence of symptomatic POP than other racial or ethnic groups in the United States [14, 58]. In a prospective cohort study of 2270 women, the risk in Latina and white women for POP was four- to fivefold higher than in African-American women [58]. In contrast, other studies have found no relationship between POP and race or ethnicity [59]. In a cadaveric study, Zacharin [60] reported that Chinese women have stronger and thicker pubourethral ligaments, endopelvic fascia, and endopelvic attachment to the obturator fascia compared to Caucasian women. More recently, Dietz [61] confirmed these results using pelvic floor ultrasound. The reasons for these ethnic differences are unclear; however, some evidence indicates that African-American women have smaller pelvic outlets than those of European descent [12].

2.10 Connective Tissue Disorders

It has been demonstrated that young women with POP are more likely to have connective or neurological tissue diseases and congenital abnormalities [62]. For example, women with Marfan or Ehlers-Danlos syndrome have high rates of POP. Intrinsic joint hypermobility is another well-recognised connective tissue disease that is associated with pelvic descent [63, 64]. This finding supports the hypothesised aetiological role of connective tissue disorders as a factor in the pathogenesis of this conditions [65, 66].

2.11 Constipation

Chronic constipation is a risk factor for POP, likely due to repetitive increases in intraabdominal pressure [67, 68]. Individuals with stage 2 or greater pelvic organ prolapse had an increased risk of constipation (OR 3.9; 95% CI: 1.4–11.9) compared to women with stage 0 or 1 prolapse [69]. However, findings of larger studies have disputed this association [67, 70]. Data conflict regarding whether the risk of prolapse is increased in women with occupations that involve heavy lifting [71].

2.12 Previous Surgery

Although hysterectomy might increase the risk of subsequent POP, prolapse symptoms typically develop many years after this procedure [66]. According to Mant et al., in the Oxford Family Planning study, the incidence of prolapse which required surgical correction following hysterectomy was 3.6 per 1000 person-years of risk. The cumulative risk rises from 1% 3 years after a hysterectomy to 5% 15 years after hysterectomy. The risk of prolapse following hysterectomy is 5.5 times higher (95% CI 3.1–9.7) in women whose initial hysterectomy was for genital prolapse as opposed to other reasons.

Contrary to findings of many other studies, the prevalence of prolapse in women with a uterus in the Women's Health Initiative was slightly higher than for those who had undergone hysterectomy, suggesting that previous prolapse of pelvic organs might have been repaired at the time of the procedure in this study population [14, 66].

References

1. Wei JT, DeLancey JOL. Functional anatomy of the pelvic floor and lower urinary tract. Clin Obstet Gynecol. 2004;47(1):3–17.
2. DeLancey JOL. Anatomy and biomechanics of genital prolapse. Clin Obstet Gynecol. 1993;36(4):897–909.
3. Haylen BT, de Ridder D, Freeman RM, Swift SE, Berghmans B, Lee J, Monga A, Petri E, Rizk DE, Sand PK, Schaer GN. An International Urogynecological Association (IUGA)/ International Continence Society (ICS) Joint Report on the Terminology for Female Pelvic Floor Dysfunction. Neurourol Urodyn. 2010;29:4–20.
4. Hall AF, Theofrastous JP, Cundiff GW, et al. Interobserver and intraobserver reliability of the proposed International Continence Society, Society of Gynecologic Surgeons, and American Urogynecologic Society pelvic organ prolapse classification system. Am J Obstet Gynecol. 1996;175:1467.
5. Treszezamsky AD, Rascoff L, Shahryarinejad A, Vardy MD. Use of pelvic organ prolapse staging systems in published articles of selected specialized journals. Int Urogynecol J. 2010;21:359.
6. Vierhout ME, Stoutjesdijk J, Spruijt JA. comparison of preoperative and intraoperative evaluation of patients undergoing pelvic reconstructive surgery for pelvic organ prolapse using the Pelvic Organ Prolapse Quantification System. Int Urogynecol J Pelvic Floor Dysfunct. 2006;17:46.
7. Swift S, Morris S, McKinnie V, Freeman R, Petri E, Scotti RJ, Dwyer P. Validation of a simplified technique for using the POPQ pelvic organ prolapse classification system. Int Urogynecol J Pelvic Floor Dysfunct. 2006;17(6):615–20.
8. Milsom I, Altman D, Cartwright R, Lapitan MC, Nelson R, Sillén U, Tikkinen K. Epidemiology of Urinary Incontinence (UI) and other Lower Urinary Tract Symptoms (LUTS), Pelvic Organ Prolapse (POP) and Anal Incontinence (AI)—5th ICI. Paris: Health Publication Ltd; 2013.
9. Serati M, Braga A, Bogani G, Roberti Maggiore UL, Sorice P, Ghezzi F, Salvatore S. Iliococcygeus fixation for the treatment of apical vaginal prolapse: efficacy and safety at 5 years of follow-up. Int Urogynecol J. 2015;26(7):1007–12.
10. Maher C, Baessler K, Barber M et al. Surgical management of pelvic organ prolapse. In: Abrams C, Khoury W, editors. 5th ICI. Paris: Health Publication Ltd.
11. Barber MD, Maher C. Epidemiology and outcome assessment of pelvic organ prolapse. Int Urogynecol J. 2013;24:1783.
12. Nygaard I, Barber MD, Burgio KL, et al. Prevalence of symptomatic pelvic floor disorders in US women. JAMA. 2008;300:1311.
13. Barber MD, Walters MF, Bump RC. Short forms of two condition-specific quality-of-life questionnaires for women with pelvic floor disorders (PFDI-20 and PFIQ-7). Am J Obstet Gynecol. 2005;193:103–13.
14. Hendrix SL, Clark A, Nygaard I, et al. Pelvic organ prolapse in the Women's Health Initiative: gravity and gravidity. Am J Obstet Gynecol. 2002;186:1160.
15. Swift SE. The distribution of pelvic organ support in a population of female subjects seen for routine gynecologic health care. Am J Obstet Gynecol. 2000;183:277.
16. Chow D, Rodrìguez LV. Epidemiology and prevalence of pelvic organ prolapse. Curr Opin Urol. 2013;23:293–8.
17. Neuman M, Lavy Y. Conservation of the prolapsed uterus is a valid option: medium term results of a prospective comparative study with the posterior intravaginal slingoplasty operation. Int Urogynecol J Pelvic Floor Dysfunct. 2007;18(8):889–93.
18. Bradley CS, Zimmerman MB, Qi Y, et al. Natural history of pelvic organ prolapse in post-menopausal women. Obstet Gynecol. 2007;109:848.
19. Luber KM, Boero S, Choe JY. The demographics of pelvic floor disorders: current observations and future projections. Am J Obstet Gynecol. 2001;184(7):1496–501. discussion 1501–1503.
20. Shah AD, Kohli N, Rajan SS, Hoyte L. The age distribution, rates, and types of surgery for pelvic organ prolapse in the USA. Int Urogynecol J Pelvic Floor Dysfunct. 2008;19(3):421–8.
21. Wu JM, Hundley AF, Fulton RG, Myers ER. Forecasting the prevalence of pelvic floor disorders in US women: 2010 to 2050. Obstet Gynecol. 2009;114(6):1278–83.

22. Rortveit G, Brown JS, Thom DH, Van Den Eeden SK, Creasman JM, Subak LL. Symptomatic pelvic organ prolapse: prevalence and risk factors in a population-based, racially diverse cohort. Obstet Gynecol. 2007;109(6):1396–403.
23. Handa VL, Garrett E, Hendrix S, Gold E, Robbins J. Progression and remission of pelvic organ prolapse: a longitudinal study of menopausal women. Am J Obstet Gynecol. 2004;190(1):27–32.
24. Nygaard I, Bradley C, Brandt D, Initiative W's H. Pelvic organ prolapse in older women: prevalence and risk factors. Obstet Gynecol. 2004;104(3):489–97.
25. Marchionni M, Bracco GL, Checcucci V, Carabaneanu A, Coccia EM, Mecacci F, Scarselli G. True incidence of vaginal vault prolapse. Thirteen years of experience. J Reprod Med. 1999;44(8):679–84.
26. Aigmueller T, Dungl A, Hinterholzer S, Geiss I, Riss P. An estimation of the frequency of surgery for posthysterectomy vault prolapsed. Int Urogynecol J. 2010;21:299–302.
27. Cassado Garriga J, et al. Tridimensional sonographic anatomical changes on pelvic floor muscle according to the type of delivery. Int Urogynecol J. 2011;22(8):1011–8.
28. Heilbrun ME, et al. Correlation between levator ani muscle injuries on magnetic resonance imaging and fecal incontinence, pelvic organ prolapse, and urinary incontinence in primiparous women. Am J Obstet Gynecol. 2010;202(5):488 e1–6.
29. Dietz HP, Lanzarone V. Levator trauma after vaginal delivery. Obstet Gynecol. 2005;106(4):707–12.
30. Dietz HP, Simpson JM. Levator trauma is associated with pelvic organ prolapse. Br J Obstet Gynaecol. 2008;115(8):979–84.
31. Mant J, Painter R, Vessey M. Epidemiology of genital prolapse: observations from the Oxford Family Planning Association Study. Br J Obstet Gynaecol. 1997;104:579–85.
32. Patel DA, Xu X, Thomason AD, et al. Childbirth and pelvic floor dysfunction: an epidemiologic approach to the assessment of prevention opportunities at delivery. Am J Obstet Gynecol. 2006;195:23.
33. Leijonhufvud A, et al. Risks of stress urinary incontinence and pelvic organ prolapse surgery in relation to mode of childbirth. Am J Obstet Gynecol. 2011;204(1):70 e1–7.
34. Gyhagen M, Bullarbo M, Nielsen TF, Milsom I. Prevalence and risk factors for pelvic organ prolapse 20 years after childbirth: a national cohort study in singleton primiparae after vaginal or caesarean delivery. Br J Obstet Gynaecol. 2013;120(2):152–60.
35. Rahn DD, et al. Biomechanical properties of the vaginal wall: effect of pregnancy, elastic fiber deficiency, and pelvic organ prolapse. Am J Obstet Gynecol. 2008;98(5):590 e1–6.
36. O'Boyle AL, et al. The natural history of pelvic organ support in pregnancy. Int Urogynecol J Pelvic Floor Dysfunct. 2003;14(1):46–9. discussion 49.
37. O'Boyle AL, Woodman PJ, O'Boyle JD, Davis GD, Swift SE. Pelvic organ support in nulliparous pregnant and nonpregnant women: a case control study. Am J Obstet Gynecol. 2002;187:99–102.
38. Sze EH, Sherard GB 3rd, Dolezal JM. Pregnancy, labor, delivery, and pelvic organ prolapse. Obstet Gynecol. 2002;100(5 Pt 1):981–6.
39. Chan SS, Cheung RY, Yiu AK, et al. Prevalence of levator ani muscle injury in Chinese women after first delivery. Ultrasound Obstet Gynecol. 2011;39:704–709.35.
40. Handa VL, Blomquist JL, McDermott KC, et al. Pelvic floor disorders after vaginal birth: effect of episiotomy, perineal laceration, and operative birth. Obstet Gynecol. 2012;119(2 Pt 1):233–9.
41. Uma R, Libby G, Murphy DJ. Obstetric management of a woman's first delivery and the implications for pelvic floor surgery in later life. Br J Obstet Gynaecol. 2005;112:1043–6.
42. Moalli PA, et al. Risk factors associated with pelvic floor disorders in women undergoing surgical repair. Obstet Gynecol. 2003;101(5 Pt 1):869–74.
43. Swift SE, Tate SB, Nicholas J. Correlation of symptoms with degree of pelvic organ support in a general population of women: what is pelvic organ prolapse? Am J Obstet Gynecol. 2003;189(2):372–7; discussion 377-9.
44. Swift S, Woodman P, O'Boyle A, et al. Pelvic Organ Support Study (POSST): the distribution, clinical definition, and epidemiologic condition of pelvic organ support defects. Am J Obstet Gynecol. 2005;192:795.

45. Kudish BI, Iglesia CB, Sokol RJ, et al. Effect of weight change on natural history of pelvic organ prolapse. Obstet Gynecol. 2009;113:81.
46. Daucher JA, Ellison RE, Lowder JL. Pelvic support and urinary function improve in women after surgically induced weight reduction. Female Pelvic Med Reconstr Surg. 2010;16:263.
47. Boyles SH, Weber AM, Meyn L. Procedures for pelvic organ prolapse in the United States, 1979–1997. Am J Obstet Gynecol. 2003;188(1):108–15.
48. Shah AD, Kohli N, Rajan SS, Hoyte L. The age distribution, rates, and types of surgery for pelvic organ prolapse in the USA. Int Urogynecol J Pelvic Floor Dysfunct. 2008;19(3):421–8.
49. Chiaffarino F, et al. Reproductive factors, family history, occupation and risk of urogenital prolapse. Eur J Obstet Gynecol Reprod Biol. 1999;82(1):63–7.
50. Jack GS, et al. Familial transmission of genitovaginal prolapse. Int Urogynecol J Pelvic Floor Dysfunct. 2006;17(5):498–501.
51. Altman D, et al. Genetic influence on stress urinary incontinence and pelvic organ prolapse. Eur Urol. 2008;54(4):918–22.
52. Buchsbaum GM, et al. Pelvic organ prolapse in nulliparous women and their parous sisters. Obstet Gynecol. 2006;108(6):1388–93.
53. Allen-Brady K, et al. Identification of six loci associated with pelvic organ prolapse using genome-wide association analysis. Obstet Gynecol. 2011;118(6):1345–53.
54. Nikolova G, et al. Sequence variant in the laminin gamma1 (LAMC1) gene associated with familial pelvic organ prolapse. Hum Genet. 2007;120(6):847–56.
55. Visco AG, Yuan L. Differential gene expression in pubococcygeus muscle from patients with pelvic organ prolapse. Am J Obstet Gynecol. 2003;189(1):102–12.
56. Connell KA, et al. HOXA11 is critical for development and maintenance of uterosacral ligaments and deficient in pelvic prolapse. J Clin Invest. 2008;118(3):1050–5.
57. Kim S, Harvey MA, Johnston S. A review of the epidemiology and pathophysiology of pelvic floor dysfunction: do racial differences matter? J Obstet Gynaecol Can. 2005;27(3):251–9.
58. Whitcomb EL, Rortveit G, Brown JS, et al. Racial differences in pelvic organ prolapse. Obstet Gynecol. 2009;114:1271.
59. Sears CL, Wright J, O'Brien J, et al. The racial distribution of female pelvic floor disorders in an equal access health care system. J Urol. 2009;181:187.
60. Zacharin RF. Abdominoperineal urethral suspension: a ten-year experience in the management of recurrent stress incontinence of urine. Obstet Gynecol. 1977;50(1):1–8.
61. Dietz HP. Do Asian women have less pelvic organ mobility than Caucasians? Int Urogynecol J Pelvic Floor Dysfunct. 2003;14(4):250–3; discussion 253.
62. Strohbehn K, Jakary JA, Delancey JO. Pelvic organ prolapse in young women. Obstet Gynecol. 1997;90(1):33–6.
63. Al-Rawi ZS, Al-Rawi ZT. Joint hypermobility in women with genital prolapse. Lancet. 1982;1(8287):1439–41.
64. Norton PA, et al. Genitourinary prolapse and joint hypermobility in women. Obstet Gynecol. 1995;85(2):225–8.
65. Carley ME, Schaffer J. Urinary incontinence and pelvic organ prolapse in women with Marfan or Ehlers Danlos syndrome. Am J Obstet Gynecol. 2000;182(5):1021–3.
66. Koelbl H, et al. Pathophysiology of urinary incontinence, faecal incontinence and pelvic organ prolapse. In: Abrams C, Khoury W, editors. 5th ICI. Paris: Health Publication Ltd.
67. Weber AM, Walters MD, Ballard LA, et al. Posterior vaginal prolapse and bowel function. Am J Obstet Gynecol. 1998;179:1446.
68. Spence-Jones C, Kamm MA, Henry MM, Hudson CN. Bowel dysfunction: a pathogenic factor in uterovaginal prolapse and urinary stress incontinence. Br J Obstet Gynaecol. 1994;101:147.
69. Arya LA, et al. Pelvic organ prolapse, constipation, and dietary fiber intake in women: a case-control study. Am J Obstet Gynecol. 2005;192(5):1687–91.
70. Jelovsek, J.E., et al., Functional bowel and anorectal disorders in patients with pelvic organ prolapse and incontinence. Am J Obstet Gynecol, 2005. 193(6): p. 2105-2111.4
71. Jørgensen S, Hein HO, Gyntelberg F. Heavy lifting at work and risk of genital prolapse and herniated lumbar disc in assistant nurses. Occup Med (Lond). 1994;44:47.

Concomitant Functional Disorders in Genito-Urinary Prolapse

3

Enrico Finazzi Agrò and Daniele Bianchi

3.1 Concomitant Functional Disorders in Genito-Urinary Prolapse

Genito-urinary prolapse can present with functional disorders that sometimes worsen with physical activity or abdominal strain. The most recent guidelines distinguish between symptoms related to urinary incontinence, bladder storage, sensory function, voiding or postvoiding, pelvic organ prolapse, sexual dysfunction, anorectal dysfunction and lower urinary tract or other pelvic pain. Urinary incontinence itself is defined as an involuntary loss of urine [1]. For a complete definition list, see Table 3.1.

3.2 Some General Considerations

Storage symptoms have a heavier impact on quality of life than do voiding symptoms [2]. In particular, some studies of overactive bladder syndrome (OAB) have reported a prevalence of 12% in both men and women, and OAB diminished the health-related quality of life (HRQL), emotional well-being and work productivity. A weak stream, split stream, nocturia, urgency, stress urinary incontinence, coital incontinence and incomplete emptying were significantly associated with anxiety in women [3]. The association of LUTS with anxiety and depression raises the issue of public healthcare costs, thereby requiring effort towards an early diagnosis and proper early treatment.

E. Finazzi Agrò (✉) · D. Bianchi
Department of Experimental Medicine and Surgery, University of Rome Tor Vergata, Rome, Italy

UOSD Functional Urology, Policlinico Tor Vergata, Rome, Italy
e-mail: finazzi.agro@med.uniroma2.it

© Springer International Publishing AG, part of Springer Nature 2018
V. Li Marzi, M. Serati (eds.), *Management of Pelvic Organ Prolapse*,
Urodynamics, Neurourology and Pelvic Floor Dysfunctions,
https://doi.org/10.1007/978-3-319-59195-7_3

Table 3.1 Definitions of symptoms related to female pelvic floor dysfunctions [1]

Urinary incontinence symptoms
Stress urinary incontinence
Complaint of involuntary loss of urine on effort or physical exertion or on coughing or sneezing
Urgency urinary incontinence
Complaint of involuntary loss of urine associated with urgency
Postural urinary incontinence
Postural urinary incontinence has been recently introduced to describe the loss of urine secondary to the change of body position
Nocturnal enuresis
Complaint of urine loss while sleeping
Mixed urinary incontinence
Involuntary loss of urine associated with urgency as well as with effort or physical exertion or on sneezing or coughing
Continuous urinary incontinence
Complaint of continuous involuntary loss of urine
Insensible urinary incontinence
Insensible urinary incontinence has been recently defined as a loss of urine with the patient unaware of how it happened
Coital incontinence
Coital incontinence is the involuntary loss of urine during coitus occurring either at penetration/intromission or orgasm
Bladder storage symptoms
Increased daytime urinary frequency
Increased daytime urinary frequency is the need to perform micturition more frequently during the waking hours than previously reported by the patient
Nocturia
Nocturia is the need to interrupt sleep in order to micturate (each voiding is preceded and followed by sleep)
Urgency
A sudden, compelling desire to pass urine which is difficult to defer
Overactive bladder syndrome (OAB syndrome)
Overactive bladder (OAB) syndrome consists of urinary urgency, usually along with frequency and nocturia, with or without urgency urinary incontinence, in the absence of urinary tract infections or any other obvious pathology
This condition deserves an accurate differential diagnosis to exclude neurologic disorders and with bladder cancer, as these can occasionally present with urgency
Sensory symptoms
Increased bladder sensation
Complaint that the desire to void during bladder filling occurs earlier or is more persistent than previously experienced (this differs from urgency by the fact that micturition can be postponed despite the desire to void)
Reduced bladder sensation
Complaint that the definite desire to void occurs later than previously experienced, despite an awareness that the bladder is filling
Absent bladder sensation
Complaint of both the absence of the sensation of bladder filling and a definite desire to void

Table 3.1 (continued)

Voiding or postvoiding symptoms

Hesitancy
Complaint of a delay in starting micturition

Slow stream
Complaint of a urinary stream perceived as slower than previous performances or in comparison with others

Intermittency
Complaint of urine flow that stops and starts on one or more occasions during voiding

Straining to void
Complaint of the need to make an intensive effort, such as abdominal straining, the valsalva manoeuvre or suprapubic pressure, in order to start, maintain or improve the urinary stream

Spraying (splitting) of the urinary stream
Complaint that the urine passage is a spray or split rather than a single discrete stream

Feeling of incomplete bladder emptying
Complaint that the bladder does not feel empty after micturition

Need to immediately re-void
Complaint that further micturition is necessary soon after passing urine

Post-micturition leakage
Complaint of a further involuntary passage of urine following the completion of micturition

Position-dependent micturition
Complaint of having to take specific positions to be able to micturate spontaneously or to improve bladder emptying

Dysuria
Complaint of burning or other discomfort during micturition, either intrinsic to the lower urinary tract or external (e.g. vulvar dysuria)

Urinary retention
Complaint of the inability to pass urine despite persistent effort

Pelvic organ prolapse symptoms

Vaginal bulging
The sensation of a "bulge" or "something coming down" towards or through the vaginal introitus. It can be seen or detected on palpation by the patient

Pelvic pressure
Complaint of increased heaviness or dragging in the suprapubic and/or pelvic area

Bleeding and infections
Complaint of vaginal bleeding, discharge or infection in relation to an ulceration of the prolapse

Splinting/digitations
Complaint of the need for digital replacement of the prolapse or for application of manual pressure to the vagina or perineum (splinting) or to the vagina or rectum (digitation) to assist in voiding or defaecation

Low backache
Complaint of low, sacral (or "period-like") backache associated temporally with pelvic organ prolapse (POP)

3.3 A Glance at Overactive Bladder Syndrome (OAB) Treatment

According to its definition, OAB is classified as "dry" or "wet", depending on the absence or presence of urinary incontinence, respectively. OAB can present as a primary condition or associated with pelvic organ prolapse (POP) [4]. The first-line treatment for OAB consists of lifestyle and behavioural modifications, such as reducing body weight, eliminating smoking and progressively trying to prolong the interval between each micturition [5]. Obesity, in particular, is a proven risk factor for POP [6]. In any case, medical therapy, based on antimuscarinic drugs or on the more recent β3-agonists, is usually prescribed in clinical practice [7–9]. The choice between the two drug categories is based on both specific urologic features and general conditions [10]. A decrease in bladder voiding efficiency and an increase in postvoid residual urine are possible side effects of antimuscarinic agents, whilst β3-agonists (e.g. mirabegron) show no effects on these parameters. Typical antimuscarinic side effects, such as constipation and dry mouth, are also not typically associated with β3-agonists. However, β3-agonists are not recommended for patients with uncontrolled hypertension.

In addition to medical therapy, pelvic floor rehabilitation should be encouraged in patients who complain of urinary incontinence. Exercises should consist of pelvic floor muscle training, to improve muscle activity and to reduce OAB symptoms [11–14]. OAB can also be successfully treated by means of posterior tibial nerve stimulation [15–18] or sacral nerve stimulation [19]. One more treatment option for detrusor overactivity consists of endoscopic infiltration of the bladder wall with onabotulinum toxin A at the standard dosage of 100 UI. This treatment has proven efficacy in patients who do not respond to antimuscarinics, although it usually needs to be repeated within 6–12 months [20]. Topical oestrogen therapy is also used for OAB [21].

An association between OAB and POP was indicated in one study that showed a reduced efficacy of tolterodine (4 mg) in women with OAB and anterior vaginal wall prolapse when compared with women complaining of OAB not associated with prolapse [22]. A resolution of detrusor overactivity (DO) is reported in about two thirds of patients presenting with POP and concomitant DO after prolapse repair [23]. By contrast, other studies have reported de novo OAB symptoms after prolapse surgery in 5–6% at the 6–35 month follow-up [24]. Thus, as a general rule, the absence of bothersome OAB symptoms before POP surgery could be assumed as the best predictor for the absence of post-operative OAB symptoms [24].

3.4 Treatment of Stress Urinary Incontinence

Pelvic organ prolapse can be associated with stress urinary incontinence (SUI). About 25% of patients who are continent prior to prolapse surgery complain of urinary incontinence following prolapse repair [25]. Adding a bladder neck suspension at the time of abdominal prolapse repair reduces the risk of post-opera-tive SUI [26]. For this reason, some surgeons have started to add a midurethral sling at the time of prolapse surgery in order to reduce the rate of post-operative SUI, although this procedure may be associated with a higher occurrence of adverse events [25]. Other strategies include the options of adding a midurethral sling only in women presenting with urinary incontinence during preoperative cough testing or even placing a midurethral sling at a second time but only in patients showing SUI after prolapse repair.

Some authors have confirmed a reduction in the rate of urinary incontinence at 3 months after prolapse surgery by the addition of a midurethral sling in patients with a positive prolapse reduction stress test before surgery. However, this differ-ence seems to decline over the time, by 12 months of follow-up [25]. A total of 6.3 asymptomatic patients need to have prophylactic slings placed to prevent just one woman from presenting with SUI. Thus, at the moment, whether the benefits of this strategy outweigh the risks of adverse events remains unclear.

3.5   Detrusor Underactivity

The terms "detrusor underactivity" and "detrusor contractility" were introduced in 2002 to describe reductions in maximum flow rate and detrusor pressure, although these terms and their related signs are still surrounded by ambiguity and confusion [27]. The occurrence of urinary retention after urogynaecological surgery has been estimated to range between 2.5 and 43.0% [28]. Many factors have been proposed, but poor detrusor contraction seems to have a key role. On the other hand, even a mild prolapse correction could lead to symptom improvement, given the reduction of compressive forces proximal to an intact retrovesical angle [29].

3.6   Role of Urodynamic Tests

The role of invasive urodynamic tests in the preoperative evaluation for POP is still under debate in the literature. Regardless, these tests should be considered essential in many cases, depending on the patient's clinical features [30]. Urodynamic data are also valuable as they can be used to provide the patient with proper counselling prior to POP surgery [31, 32].

3.7   Coital Incontinence

Coital urinary incontinence is a frequently underreported but bothersome condition. Its incidence is reported to range between 10 and 27%. Some evidence suggests an association between urinary leakage at penetration and urodynamic stress inconti-nence, as well as urinary leakage during orgasm and DO. After a urodynamic diag-nosis, coital urinary incontinence at penetration can be cured in more than 80% of cases by surgery for urodynamic stress incontinence, whilst the form of coital incontinence during orgasm is curable by antimuscarinic treatment in about 60% of cases when associated with DO [33].

3.8   Symptoms of Sexual Dysfunction

Symptoms of sexual dysfunction can be associated with POP and can be classified as reported below, according to the International Continence Society/International Urogynecological Association (ICS/IUGA) standardisation of terminology [1].

3.8.1   Dyspareunia

This is a complaint of persistent or recurrent pain or discomfort associated with attempted or complete vaginal penetration. It can be divided into superficial (or introital) and deep dyspareunia in relation with the level of vaginal penetration.

3.8.2   Obstructed Intercourse

This is a complaint that vaginal penetration is not possible due to an obstacle.

3.8.3   Vaginal Laxity

This is a complaint of excessive vaginal laxity.

Up to 64% of women undergoing a urogynaecological evaluation complain of sexual dysfunction [34]. Overall, sexual function improves after surgery for stress incontinence or POP [35], but there is a need of more studies, including randomised clinical trials, specially regarding surgery with meshes, to elucidate the potential differences due to mesh features.

3.9   Lower Urinary Tract Pain and/or Other Pelvic Pain

Pain can be associated with POP. Pain can be classified as reported below, according to the ICS/IUGA standardisation of terminology [1].

3.9.1   Bladder Pain

This is a complaint of suprapubic or retropubic pain, pressure or discomfort, related to the bladder, and usually increasing with bladder filling. It may persist or be relieved after voiding.

3.9.2 Urethral Pain

This is a complaint of pain felt in the urethra, and the woman indicates the urethra as the site.

3.9.3 Vulval Pain

This is a complaint of pain felt in and around the vulva.

3.9.4 Vaginal Pain

This is a complaint of pain felt internally within the vagina, above the introitus.

3.9.5 Perineal Pain

This is a complaint of pain felt between the posterior fourchette (posterior lip of the introitus) and the anus.

3.9.6 Pelvic Pain

This is a complaint of pain perceived to arise in the pelvis but not associated with symptoms suggestive of lower urinary tract, sexual, bowel or gynaecological dysfunction. It is less well defined than the above types of localised pain.

3.9.7 Cyclical (Menstrual) Pelvic Pain

Cyclical pelvic pain related to menses raises the possibility of a gynaecological cause.

3.9.8 Pudendal Neuralgia

- Burning vaginal or vulval (anywhere between the anus and clitoris) pain associated with tenderness over the course of the pudendal nerves. Recently, five essential criteria (Nantes criteria) have been proposed for the diagnosis of pudendal neuropathy [36]: (a) pain in the anatomical region of pudendal innervation, (b) pain that is worse with sitting, (c) no waking at night with pain, (d) no sensory deficit on examination, and (e) relief of symptoms with a pudendal block.
- Chronic lower urinary tract and/or other pelvic pain syndromes.

3.10   Lower Urinary Tract Infections

Urinary tract infections may be observed in a pelvic organ prolapse. Some possibly related definitions include [1]:

- Urinary tract infection (UTI): Scientific diagnosis of a UTI is the finding of microbiological evidence of significant bacteriuria and pyuria that is usually accompanied by symptoms such as increased bladder sensation, urgency, frequency, dysuria, urgency urinary incontinence and/or pain in the lower urinary tract.
- Recurrent urinary tract infections (UTIs): At least three symptomatic and medically diagnosed UTIs in the previous 12 months. The previous UTI(s) should have resolved prior to a further UTI being diagnosed.
- Other related history: for example, haematuria or catheterisation.

References

1. Haylen BT, de Ridder D, Freeman RM, Swift SE, Berghmans B, Lee J, Monga A, Petri E, Rizk DE, Sand PK, Schaer GN, Association, International Urogynecological and Society, International Continence. An International Urogynecological Association (IUGA)/ International Continence Society (ICS) joint report on the terminology for female pelvic floor dysfunction. Neurourol Urodyn. 2010;29(1):4–20. https://doi.org/10.1002/nau.20798.
2. Coyne KS, Sexton CC, Thompson CL, Milsom I, Irwin D, Kopp ZS, Chapple CR, Kaplan S, Tubaro A, Aiyer LP, Wein AJ. The prevalence of lower urinary tract symptoms (LUTS) in the USA, the UK and Sweden: results from the epidemiology of LUTS (EpiLUTS) study. BJU Int. 2009;104(3):352–60. https://doi.org/10.1111/j.1464-410X.2009.08427.x. Epub 2009 Mar 5.
3. Lim JR, Bak CW, Lee JB. Comparison of anxiety between patients with mixed incontinence and those with stress urinary incontinence. Scand J Urol Nephrol. 2007;41(5):403–6. Epub 2007 Apr 13.
4. de Boer TA, Salvatore S, Cardozo L, Chapple C, Kelleher C, van Kerrebroeck P, Kirby MG, Koelbl H, Espuna-Pons M, Milsom I, Tubaro A, Wagg A, Vierhout ME. Pelvic organ prolapse and overactive bladder. Neurourol Urodyn. 2010;29(1):30–9. https://doi.org/10.1002/nau.20858.
5. Willis-Gray MG, Dieter AA, Geller EJ. Evaluation and management of overactive bladder: strategies for optimizing care. Res Rep Urol. 2016;8:113–22. https://doi.org/10.2147/RRU.S93636.eCollection.2016.
6. Giri A, Hartmann KE, Hellwege JN, Velez Edwards DR, Edwards TL. Obesity and pelvic organ prolapse: a systematic review and meta-analysis of observational studies. Am J Obstet Gynecol. 2017. pii: S0002-9378(17)30174-6. https://doi.org/10.1016/j.ajog.2017.01.039. [Epub ahead of print].
7. Andersson KE. Antimuscarinics for treatment of overactive bladder. Lancet Neurol. 2004;3(1):46–53.
8. Thiagamoorthy G, Kotes S, Zacchè M, Cardozo L. The efficacy and tolerability of mirabegron, a β3 adrenoceptor agonist, in patients with symptoms of overactive bladder. Ther Adv Urol. 2016;8(1):38–46. https://doi.org/10.1177/1756287215614237.
9. Olivera CK, Meriwether K, El-Nashar S, et al. Nonantimuscarinic treatment for overactive bladder: a systematic review. Am J Obstet Gynecol. 2016;215(1):34–57. https://doi.org/10.1016/j.ajog.2016.01.156. Epub 2016 Feb 4.

10. Wagg A, Nitti VW, Kelleher C, Castro-Diaz D, Siddiqui E, Berner T. Oral pharmacotherapy for overactive bladder in older patients: mirabegron as a potential alternative to antimuscarinics. Curr Med Res Opin. 2016;32(4):621–38. https://doi.org/10.1185/03007995.2016.114980 6. Epub 2016 Feb 17.
11. Voorham JC, De Wachter S, Van den Bos TW, Putter H, Lycklama À, Nijeholt GA, Voorham-van der Zalm PJ. The effect of EMG biofeedback assisted pelvic floor muscle therapy on symptoms of the overactive bladder syndrome in women: a randomized controlled trial. Neurourol Urodyn. 2016. https://doi.org/10.1002/nau.23180. [Epub ahead of print].
12. Di Gangi Herms AM, Veit R, Reisenauer C, Herms A, Grodd W, Enck P, Stenzl A, Birbaumer N. Functional imaging of stress urinary incontinence. NeuroImage. 2006;29(1):267–75. Epub 2005 Sep 8.
13. Lamin E, Parrillo LM, Newman DK, Smith AL. Pelvic floor muscle training: underutilization in the USA. Curr Urol Rep. 2016;17(2):10. https://doi.org/10.1007/s11934-015-0572-0.
14. Braekken IH, Majida M, Engh ME, Bø K. Can pelvic floor muscle training reverse pelvic organ prolapse and reduce prolapse symptoms? An assessor-blinded, randomized, controlled trial. Am J Obstet Gynecol. 2010;203(2):170.e1–7. https://doi.org/10.1016/j.ajog.2010.02.037. Epub 2010 May 1.
15. Peters KM, Carrico DJ, Wooldridge LS, Miller CJ, MacDiarmid SA. Percutaneous tibial nerve stimulation for the long-term treatment of overactive bladder: 3-year results of the STEP study. J Urol. 2013;189(6):2194–201. https://doi.org/10.1016/j.juro.2012.11.175. Epub 2012 Dec 3.
16. Gaziev G, Topazio L, Iacovelli V, Asimakopoulos A, Di Santo A, De Nunzio C, Finazzi-Agrò E. Percutaneous tibial nerve stimulation (PTNS) efficacy in the treatment of lower urinary tract dysfunctions: a systematic review. BMC Urol. 2013;13:61. https://doi.org/10.1186/1471-2490-13-61.
17. Burton C, Sajja A, Latthe PM. Effectiveness of percutaneous posterior tibial nerve stimulation for overactive bladder: a systematic review and meta-analysis. Neurourol Urodyn. 2012;31(8):1206–16. https://doi.org/10.1002/nau.22251. Epub 2012 May 11.
18. Vandoninck V, van Balken MR, Finazzi Agrò E, Petta F, Micali F, Heesakkers JP, Debruyne FM, Kiemeney LA, Bemelmans BL. Percutaneous tibial nerve stimulation in the treatment of overactive bladder: urodynamic data. Neurourol Urodyn. 2003;22(3):227–32.
19. Gupta P, Ehlert MJ, Sirls LT, Peters KM. Percutaneous tibial nerve stimulation and sacral neuromodulation: an update. Curr Urol Rep. 2015;16(2):4. https://doi.org/10.1007/s11934-014-0479-1.
20. Nitti VW, Dmochowski R, Herschorn S, Sand P, Thompson C, Nardo C, Yan X, Haag-Molkenteller C, EMBARK Study Group. OnabotulinumtoxinA for the treatment of patients with overactive bladder and urinary incontinence: results of a phase 3, randomized, placebo controlled trial. J Urol. 2017;197(2S):S216–23. https://doi.org/10.1016/j.juro.2016.10.109. Epub 2016 Dec 22.
21. Robinson D, Cardozo L, Milsom I, Pons ME, Kirby M, Koelbl H, Vierhout M. Oestrogens and overactive bladder. Neurourol Urodyn. 2014;33(7):1086–91. https://doi.org/10.1002/nau.22464. Epub 2013 Jul 19.
22. Salvatore S, Serati M, Ghezzi F, Uccella S, Cromi A, Bolis P. Efficacy of tolterodine in women with detrusor overactivity and anterior vaginal wall prolapse: is it the same? BJOG. 2007;114(11):1436–8. Epub 2007 Sep 17.
23. Nguyen JK, Bhatia NN. Resolution of motor urge incontinence after surgical repair of pelvic organ prolapse. J Urol. 2001;166(6):2263–6.
24. de Boer TA, Kluivers KB, Withagen MI, Milani AL, Vierhout ME. Predictive factors for overactive bladder symptoms after pelvic organ prolapse surgery. Int Urogynecol J. 2010;21(9):1143–9. https://doi.org/10.1007/s00192-010-1152-y. Epub 2010 Apr 24.
25. Wei JT, Nygaard I, Richter HE, Nager CW, Barber MD, Kenton K, Amundsen CL, Schaffer J, Meikle SF, Spino C, Pelvic Floor Disorders Network. A midurethral sling to reduce incontinence after vaginal prolapse repair. N Engl J Med. 2012;366(25):2358–67. https://doi.org/10.1056/NEJMoa1111967.
26. Brubaker L, Cundiff GW, Fine P, Nygaard I, Richter HE, Visco AG, Zyczynski H, Brown MB, Weber AM, Pelvic Floor Disorders Network. Abdominal sacrocolpopexy with Burch colposuspension to reduce urinary stress incontinence. N Engl J Med. 2006;354(15):1557–66.

27. Osman NI, Chapple CR, Abrams P, Dmochowski R, Haab F, Nitti V, Koelbl H, van Kerrebroeck P, Wein AJ. Detrusor underactivity and the underactive bladder: a new clinical entity? A review of current terminology, definitions, epidemiology, aetiology, and diagnosis. Eur Urol. 2014;65(2):389–98. https://doi.org/10.1016/j.eururo.2013.10.015. Epub 2013 Oct 26.
28. Geller EJ. Prevention and management of postoperative urinary retention after urogynecologic surgery. Int J Womens Health. 2014;6:829–38. https://doi.org/10.2147/IJWH.S55383. eCollection 2014.
29. Fletcher SG, Haverkorn RM, Yan J, Lee JJ, Zimmern PE, Lemack GE. Demographic and urodynamic factors associated with persistent OAB after anterior compartment prolapse repair. Neurourol Urodyn. 2010;29(8):1414–8. https://doi.org/10.1002/nau.20881.
30. Serati M, Topazio L, Bogani G, Costantini E, Pietropaolo A, Palleschi G, Carbone A, Soligo M, Del Popolo G, Li Marzi V, Salvatore S, Finnazzi AE. Urodynamics useless before surgery for female stress urinary incontinence: are you sure? Results from a multicenter single nation database. Neurourol Urodyn. 2016;35(7):809–12. https://doi.org/10.1002/nau.22804. Epub 2015 Jun 9.
31. Huang L, He L, Wu SL, Sun RY, Lu D. Impact of preoperative urodynamic testing for urinary incontinence and pelvic organ prolapse on clinical management in Chinese women. J Obstet Gynaecol Res. 2016;42(1):72–6. https://doi.org/10.1111/jog.12854. Epub 2015 Nov 4.
32. Baessler K, Maher C. Pelvic organ prolapse surgery and bladder function. Pelvic organ prolapse surgery and bladder function. Int Urogynecol J. 2013;24(11):1843–52. https://doi.org/10.1007/s00192-013-2175-y.
33. Serati M, Salvatore S, Uccella S, Nappi RE, Bolis P. Female urinary incontinence during intercourse: a review on an understudied problem for women's sexuality. J Sex Med. 2009;6(1):40–8. https://doi.org/10.1111/j.1743-6109.2008.01055.x.
34. Basson R, Berman J, Burnett A, Derogatis L, Ferguson D, Fourcroy J, Goldstein I, Graziottin A, Heiman J, Laan E, Leiblum S, Padma-Nathan H, Rosen R, Segraves K, Segraves RT, Shabsigh R, Sipski M, Wagner G, Whipple B. Report of the international consensus development conference on female sexual dysfunction: definitions and classifications. J Urol. 2000;163(3):888–93.
35. Rogers RG, Kammerer-Doak D, Darrow A, Murray K, Qualls C, Olsen A, Barber M. Does sexual function change after surgery for stress urinary incontinence and/or pelvic organ prolapse? A multicenter prospective study. Am J Obstet Gynecol. 2006;195(5):e1–4.
36. Labat JJ, Riant T, Robert R, Amarenco G, Lefaucheur JP, Rigaud J. Diagnostic criteria for pudendal neuralgia by pudendal nerve entrapment (Nantes criteria). Neurourol Urodyn. 2008;27(4):306–10.

Part II

Diagnostic Work-up

Clinical Evaluation and Diagnostic Tools in Women with Prolapse

4

Fabio Del Deo, Antonio Grimaldi, and Marco Torella

A complete evaluation of pelvic organ prolapse needs the investigation of general, gynecological, and obstetric history, the inquiry of the presence of concomitant lower urinary tract symptoms, and a careful physical and instrumental examination.

1. Family history
2. Past medical history
3. Present medical history
4. Physical examination and POP quantification
5. Imaging and instrumental examination

4.1 Family History

The investigation of the family history is important to reveal a possible familiar predisposition to pelvic organ prolapse. Different studies on first-degree family members and on dizygotic and monozygotic twin pairs demonstrate the high influence of genetic factors on the onset of the prolapse [1, 2]. Different research groups are carrying out genetic studies in order to identify the polymorphisms associated with such a predisposition [3–6]. This knowledge could play an important role in the evaluation of the therapeutic choice.

F. Del Deo · A. Grimaldi · M. Torella (✉)
Department of Woman, Child and General and Specialistic Surgery,
University of Campania Luigi Vanvitelli, Caserta, Italy

© Springer International Publishing AG, part of Springer Nature 2018
V. Li Marzi, M. Serati (eds.), *Management of Pelvic Organ Prolapse*,
Urodynamics, Neurourology and Pelvic Floor Dysfunctions,
https://doi.org/10.1007/978-3-319-59195-7_4

4.2   Past Medical History

Pregnancy and childbirth, aging and menopausal status, pelvic surgery, and neurological and chronic disease are deeply linked to the development of pelvic organ prolapse.

(a) The relationship between vaginal delivery and the alteration of pelvic innervation, as well as levator ani muscle and pelvic floor ligaments, are well-founded and demonstrated by epidemiological, functional, and pathological studies; parity and birth weight are proved to be important risk factor for POP causing damage directly and indirectly to the pelvic floor support. The passage of the fetus through the pelvic hiatus plays a central role in the structural damage causing permanent stretch injury related to the deprivation of oxygen and the necrotic changes. Recently the role of pregnancy and labor on the modifications of the pelvic structures is under investigation, but the late results are still conflicting [7–12].

(b) Menopause and age itself represent important risk factor for the development of pelvic organ prolapse. The role of menopause is linked at the estrogen deficiency that may act on the connective supports. Age itself is characterized by an alteration of the normal type I–type III collagen ratio and by a physiological weakening of connectives and may be related to the loss of strength and resiliency of support and suspension structures. The combination of these factors is associated with a higher risk of pelvic organ prolapse. Studies conducted to evaluate the real impact of each condition are conflicting.

(c) Previous pelvic surgery performed for correction of prolapse is associated with a higher risk of developing prolapse compared to surgery performed for other medical indications [13].

(d) Coexisting diseases associated with a chronic increase in abdominal pressure, such as obesity, chronic respiratory diseases, and constipation, represent a risk factor for the onset and aggravation of genital prolapse. The increase in abdominal pressure places under tension pelvic floor muscles and ligamentous structures, and the chronic strain leads to a structural and progressive weakening (Fig. 4.1).

Chronic smoking too is considered a risk factor for the development of prolapse. In this case, the damage mechanism would not be associated with increased intra-abdominal pressure due to coughing but with the action of chemical substances on tissues [11, 13].

(e) Presence and severity of symptoms suggesting neurological disease. Chronic conditions such as diabetes mellitus, Parkinson's disease, or multiple sclerosis or acute conditions, such as a cerebrovascular accident, can cause a peripheral neuropathy that could affect pelvic organ support.

(f) Drug history: many drugs, frequently used in the adult population, can influence the manifestation of lower urinary tract symptoms by altering bladder capacity and sensitivity. Among these, antihypertensives, antidepressants, and antipsychotics are the most common, and taking these drugs should be thoroughly investigated.

Fig. 4.1 Action of intra-abdominal pressure on the pelvic organ supports

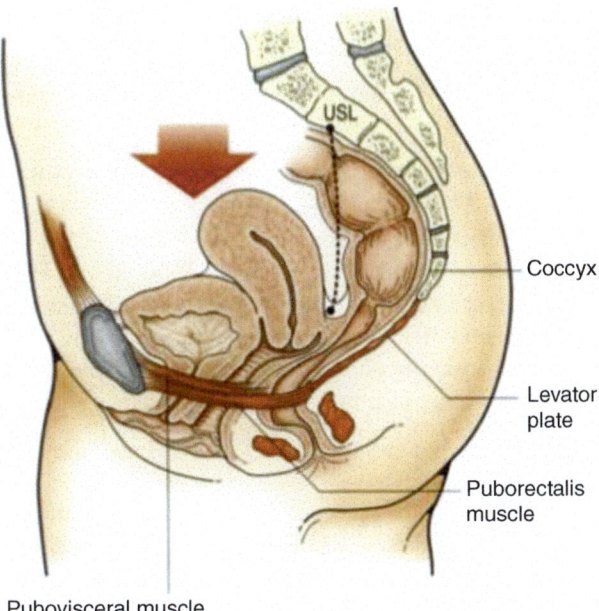

Coccyx

Levator plate

Puborectalis muscle

Pubovisceral muscle

4.3   Present Medical History

4.3.1   Clinical History

It is important to investigate the main symptoms complained by the patient, to understand their severity, the age of onset, and the progression over time. Women with pelvic organ prolapse often suffer from a wide symptomatology.

Prolapse symptoms:
- The "sense of weight" is a non-specific symptom. Frequently it appears in women with prolapse, but it is common to several diseases such as lower urinary tract infections, low back pain, and bowel disorders. It doesn't correlate with the degree of prolapse neither with a specific compartment.
- The "sense of bulge," of foreign body, is typical of patients with prolapse. It correlates to a more advanced staging, and anamnestic investigation allows the clinician to orient about the most affected district. In this case the level of protrusion, its worsening over the day, the relation to certain activities such as lifting weights or climbing stairs, the presence of pain or bleeding, the association with bladder or bowel dysfunction, and the relation with sexual and social activity should be inquired.
- Splinting/digitation: the need to manually reduce the prolapse or apply pressure to the perineum, to the vagina or to the rectum, to facilitate micturition and/or defecation.
- Low back pain related to the sensory nerves innervating the kidney and ureter, sometimes associated to the dilatation of the high urinary tract in case of high-stage prolapse hampering bladder empting.

Urinary symptoms are typical and related to the stage of prolapse:
- Storage dysfunctions:

- Stress urinary incontinence: the involuntary loss of urine, with an increase in intra-abdominal pressure, is often associated with low-stage prolapse. In case of high-stage prolapse, repositioning of the vaginal walls can unmask urinary incontinence under stress test that, in this case, is defined as "occult."
- Frequency: an increased micturition frequency; it is often related to a lower urinary tract infection, but it may also be associated with obstructive disease that causes high bladder residual volume.
- Urge urinary incontinence: a sudden and uncontrolled loss of urine associated with a feeling of urgency. Often women say not getting to the toilet in time and may lose a few drops or larger amounts of urine to a complete loss.

- Voiding dysfunctions:

- Hesitancy: the difficulty in initiating micturition; it may be associated with urethral obstruction or bladder dislocation.
- Incomplete emptying: the feeling of not having completely emptied the bladder after micturition. The displacement of the bladder or the rectum may produce concomitant ureteral compression which not allows the physiological urine emptying. This condition, if unrecognized, can cause chronic urinary tract infections for the high residuals and damage at the upper urinary tract in case of ureteral reflux.
- Intermittent flow.
- Post-micturition dribble: the loss of drops of urine after micturition is frequently associated to a urethral diverticulum but also to a cystourethrocele or detrusor overactivity.
- Straining to void: it indicates the need to make a muscle contraction in order to start and maintain the micturition; it is frequently associated with cystocele causing urethral kneeling.
- Slow stream.
- Obstruction with the need to replace the prolapse or to adopt particular positions to empty the bladder.

- Sensation dysfunctions:

- Urgency: a strong sudden desire to void
- Dysuria: painful or uncomfortable urination, typically a sharp, burning sensation
- Absent sensation

Bowel symptoms:
- Constipation is the most common defecatory symptom related to prolapse, but it represents a causal factor acting as a cause of chronic increase in abdominal pressure too. Defining its role without a specific clinical correlation could be impossible. If it is consequent to a posterior vaginal wall prolapse, physiological evacuation may be hampered or slowed by the anatomical bowel dislocation.
- Evacuation problems: in case of advanced prolapse, the patient may be forced to assume particular positions, to manually reduce the prolapse or to use the fingers in order to allow the evacuation.

Sexual symptoms:
- Vaginal bulge: the sense of protrusion. It is specific of pelvic organ prolapse, but not related to a particular compartment.
- Dyspareunia: persistent or recurrent genital pain that occurs before, during, or after sexual intercourse.
- Coital incontinence: leakage of urine during sexual intercourse, either on penetration or during orgasm. In women with anterior vaginal wall prolapse, urinary incontinence on penetration can frequently occur because of altered urethra bladder-neck anatomic ratio.

Sexual function is strictly related to genital prolapse; in some cases, intercourse is avoided for pain or mechanical difficulties, in other cases for the impact of the body image dissatisfaction that can induce women to avoid sexual intercourse causing a strong impact on couple's quality of life. This relationship is supported by the fact that after surgery sexual function improves both in women and in men [14–16].

4.3.2 Diagnostic Tools

- Questionnaires and structured interviews are validated instruments in order to investigate prolapse symptoms with a methodical approach and their impact on different areas of the quality of life. These tools consist of a series of questions that affect specific symptom domains allowing to assign a score to each response. The main difference between questionnaires and structured interviews is that the questionnaire is self-administered by the patient, while the interview is conducted by a medical figure that can insert additional questions and then assign a score based on the answers.
- Bladder diary to inquire the frequency and the volumes of micturitions and any incontinence episode.

4.4 Physical Examination and POP Quantification

The physical examination of a woman with genital prolapse begins with the inspection of vulvar skin and the assessment of the trophism of vulvovaginal mucosa. A moderate-to-severe atrophy may be observed in older women many years after menopause.

A bimanual examination should be performed to exclude pelvic masses, to assess uterine size and the presence of fibroids, and to exclude a significant post-void residual bladder volume. The presence of a urethral diverticulum should be assessed too. Ultrasound can be of great help to facilitate these investigations.

The evaluation of the degree of prolapse of the uterus (or vaginal vault) and of anterior and posterior vaginal walls is most commonly carried out in the lithotomy position. Women may be then reexamined in orthostatic position if the maximum extent of the prolapse cannot be obtained in lithotomy or if there is no correlation between reported symptoms and physical findings. In advanced prolapse the descent is clear already at rest, whereas if the prolapse is of a lesser degree, the clinician should ask the patient to cough or to perform the Valsalva maneuver, trying to reproduce the maximum protrusion of the prolapse. During the strain, the lower branch of a speculum could be useful for highlighting the vaginal compartment to evaluate.

At physical examination, it may be possible to distinguish two types of anterior vaginal wall prolapse: distension and displacement [17]. The first one is thought to be due to a midline defect (thinning or rupture) of the pubocervical fascia supporting the bladder base, with consequent loss of characteristic rugal folds of the anterior vaginal wall. In case of displacement cystocele, a pathologic detachment of the pubocervical fascia from the arcus tendineus fasciae pelvis occurs (lateral or paravaginal defect). Rugal folds are most often preserved.

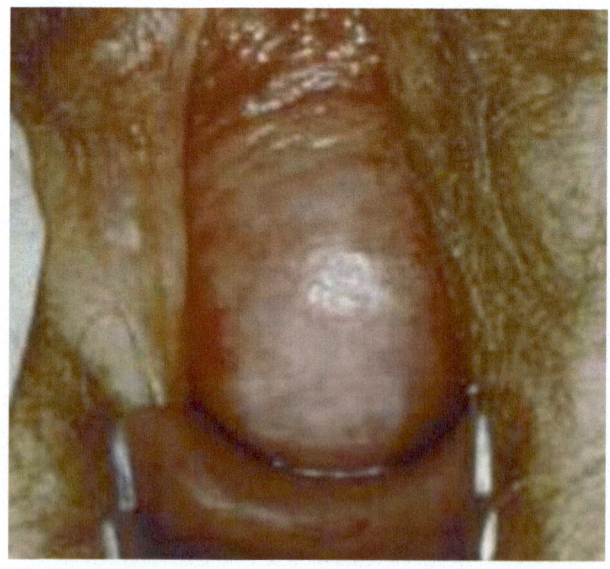

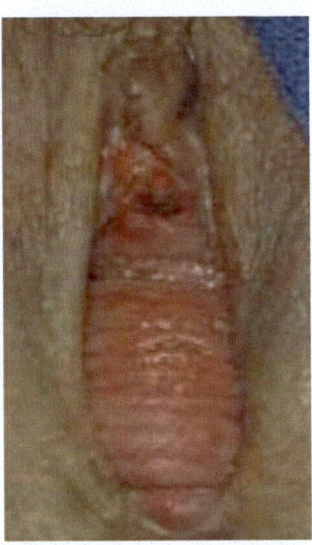

Care should be taken not to confuse the cervical elongation with a hysterocele: in this case, the walls of the cervix are so much longer that the ectocervix reaches the vulvar ostium and sometimes may leak out from the vulva. By vaginal or rectal examination, the clinician will appreciate that the uterine corpus is in its normal position and is not prolapsed. Ultrasound may also confirm the abnormal cervical length.

In the past decades, several systems for staging the degree of genital prolapse have been proposed. One of the most common grading systems was developed in 1972 by Baden and Walker and is called halfway scoring system [18]. It consists of determining the position in relation to the hymen of each single organ that is projected into the vagina (urethra, bladder, uterus or vaginal vault, posterior fornix, rectum) with the patient at maximum strain. Therefore, the terms urethrocele, cystocele, hysterocele or vault prolapse, enterocele, and rectocele are respectively used.

Prolapse severity is classified into five grades (0 to 4) for each segment. If the organ being examined remains in its original position during strain, that is, at the level of the ischial spines, it means that this organ doesn't prolapse and is classified as grade 0. If the organ under examination is positioned between the ischial spines and a midpoint between them and the hymen, we talk about grade 1 prolapse, whereas if this organ is located in a position between the latter point and the hymen, it is a second-degree descent. Prolapses extending beyond the hymenal ring represent grades 3 and 4; in particular, a third-degree prolapse does not exceed the midpoint between the hymen and the maximum protrusion of the organ (grade 4).

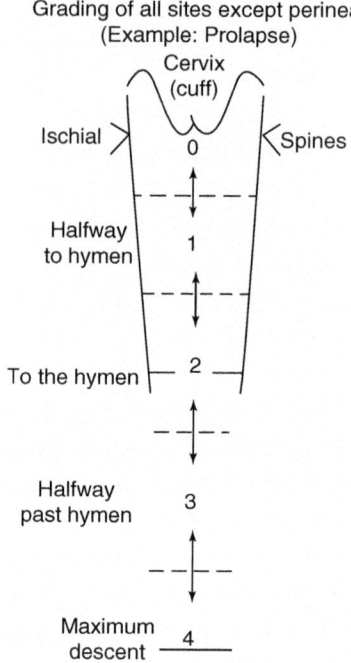

Grading of all sites except perineal
(Example: Prolapse)

The slightly used Beecham's classification, developed in 1980, is based on the degree of descent of pelvic organs in relation to the vaginal ostium [19]:

- Grade 1: prolapse does not exceed the middle third of the vagina.
- Grade 2: prolapse reaches the vaginal introitus without going over.
- Grade 3: prolapse is outside the introitus.

The major problem associated with the use of these classification systems is a certain degree of subjectivity with the consequent difficulty of comparing data between observers. Nevertheless, Baden–Walker halfway scoring system is still widely used in clinical practice for its simplicity and directness.

The need for researchers to exchange information on surgical series led to the proposal of a new method of prolapse classification called pelvic organ prolapse quantification (POP-Q) system. It was developed in 1996 and approved by the International Continence Society, American Urogynecologic Society, and Society of Gynecologic Surgeons [20]. The POP-Q advantage is to provide a very accurate prolapse staging. It consists in the quantification of the descent by identifying six specific points along the vaginal walls; these points are measured in centimeters with respect to a fixed reference point (hymenal ring), while the patient is asked to strain. The points that are located proximal to or above the hymen are expressed in centimeters preceded by the sign – (negative number), whereas those located distal to or below the hymen are expressed as positive numbers. The points located at the level of the hymenal ring are at position 0.

These landmarks are two on the anterior vaginal wall (Aa, Ba), two on the apical portion of the vagina (C, D), and two on the posterior vaginal wall (Ap, Bp). The measurements of the genital hiatus, perineal body, and total vaginal length are also detected: they are performed at rest and therefore are not preceded by any sign.

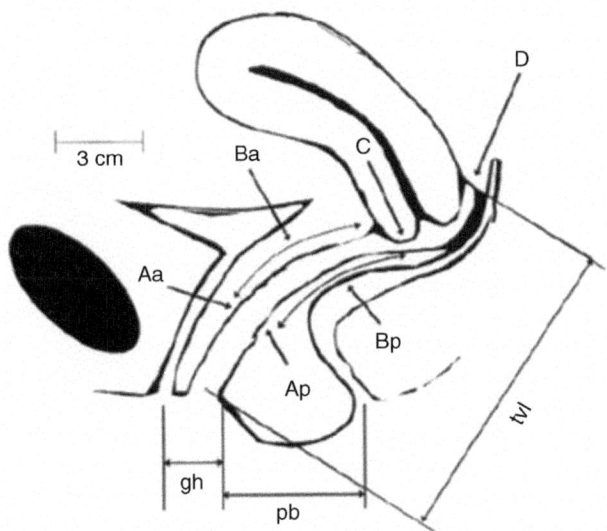

- Aa: point located along the midline of the anterior vaginal wall, 3 cm above the external urethral orifice (and the hymen); its excursion is by definition between – 3 and +3 cm. A descent of this point indicates the loss of the ureterovesical junction, and, according to some experts, it may be associated with an increased incidence of urinary stress incontinence.
- Ba: most distal point of the high portion of the anterior vaginal wall, between the anterior fornix and the point Aa; in the absence of prolapse, it is by definition located at – 3 cm. It describes the severity of the cystocele.
- C: most distal point reached by the cervix (or the vaginal vault in case of previous hysterectomy). It describes the severity of the hysterocele (or the vault prolapse).
- D: it corresponds to the posterior fornix (or Douglas pouch) and represents the insertion point of the uterosacral ligaments. It is omitted in case of previous hysterectomy. If point C is much more positive (distal) of point D, it is a cervical elongation and not a hysterocele.
- Ap: point located along the midline of the posterior vaginal wall, 3 cm above the hymen; its excursion is by definition between – 3 and +3 cm.
- Bp: most distal point of the high portion of the posterior vaginal wall, between the posterior fornix and the point Ap; in the absence of prolapse, it is by definition located at – 3 cm. It describes the severity of the rectocele.

Table 4.1 POP-Q Staging Criteria

POP-Q Staging Criteria	
Stage 0	Aa, Ap, Ba, Bp = −3 cm and C or D ≤ − (tvl − 2) cm
Stage I	Stage 0 criteria not met and leading edge < −1 cm
Stage II	Leading edge ≥ −1 cm but ≤ +1 cm
Stage III	Leading edge > +1 cm but < + (tvl − 2) cm
Stage IV	Leading edge ≥ + (tvl − 2) cm

- Gh: genital hiatus, measured from the external urethral orifice to the posterior commissure (fourchette).
- Pb: perineal body, measured from the fourchette to the anus.
- Tvl: total vaginal length, measured after the reduction of prolapse.

anterior wall	anterior wall	cervix or cuff
Aa	Ba	C
genital hiatus	perineal body	total vaginal length
gh	pb	tvl
posterior wall	posterior wall	posterior fornix
Ap	Bp	D

Even in POP-Q system, prolapse staging includes five degrees (0 to 4); see Table 4.1.

During the physical examination, it may be useful to perform the rectovaginal exam that allows the clinician to recognize a possible defect of the higher portion of the rectovaginal septum, resulting in enterocele.

Furthermore, a cough stress test with a full bladder could make objective an associated stress urinary incontinence. About 55% of women with stage II prolapse report concomitant stress incontinence. This rate decreases with increasing POP stages to 33% in women with stage IV prolapse [21]. However, if the prolapse is reduced digitally or with the help of a pessary, sponge holder, or speculum, an occult stress incontinence may be demonstrated in up to 80% of women [22–25].

In case of a positive stress test associated with a cystocele, Bonney test may be indicated because it tries to predict the likelihood of curing stress incontinence with an anterior colporrhaphy. The index and middle fingers are placed on both sides of the urethra to elevate the bladder neck while the patient is asked to cough or do a Valsalva maneuver with a full bladder: if there is no urine leakage, it means that stress incontinence is due to descent of the bladder neck and may benefit from the vaginal repair, whereas the persistence of positive stress test indicates an intrinsic sphincter deficiency. The outcome of Bonney test is, indeed, not reliable because it is difficult to standardize; therefore, this test is considered of no practical use [26].

The mobility of the urethra and bladder neck can be evaluated by inserting a sterile lubricated cotton or Dacron swab (Q-tip) into the urethra until the urethro-vesical junction. The angle formed by the distal end of the swab is measured relative to the horizontal using a goniometer during Valsalva. Urethrovesical junction hyper-mobility is defined when this angle >30°. Q-tip test may be useful to distinguish the type of stress incontinence and to indicate the most appropriate surgical procedure to perform. Therefore, a negative Q-tip test can be considered as a risk factor for failed incontinence surgery [27].

4.5   Imaging and Instrumental Examination

4.5.1   Ultrasound

In recent years, ultrasound is taking a leading role in the imaging of pelvic floor defects. The widespread availability of suitable devices, the simplicity of perfor-mance, the safety, and the noninvasive nature, as well as the cost-effectiveness, have favored a rapid spread of this technique. Different probes consent to perform trans-vaginal, abdominal, perineal/translabial, and transrectal study with a bi-, tri-, and four-dimensional reconstruction. The route that better lends to the study of genital prolapse is the transperineal one; thanks to the noninvasive investigation which does not interfere with vaginal descent. The possibility to perform a dynamic study allows an evaluation of pelvic organs at rest and after Valsalva maneuver that enable to obtain a detailed quantification of prolapse [28, 29].

4.5.1.1 Perineal/Translabial Ultrasound
Genital prolapse can be studied by perineal/translabial ultrasound. Bladder neck, cervix or cul-de-sac, and the rectal ampulla are the leading edges of anterior, cen-tral, and posterior compartment, respectively. The benchmark for the evaluation of pelvic organs descent is represented by the inferior margin of the symphysis pubis (Fig. 4.2).

To perform perineal or translabial ultrasound, patient has to gain gynecological position, and the convex probe is positioned on the perineum, between the pubis and the anal margin. Bladder has to be empty or full in relation to the parameters to be observed; rectum has to be empty in order not to affect the diagnostic accuracy. The transducer, a 3.5–6 MHz curved array, is covered with a glove or a specific device for hygienic reasons and placed on the perineum in a midsagittal plane. The pres-sure applied to the probe has to be as low as possible not to mask or underestimate organ descent. This location allows to visualize the bladder, urethra, vaginal walls, uterus, anal canal, and rectum. There is no standardization relatively to the orienta-tion of image even if most authors prefer the same applied in transvaginal methodic with the cranioventral structures on the left and the dorsocaudal on the right.

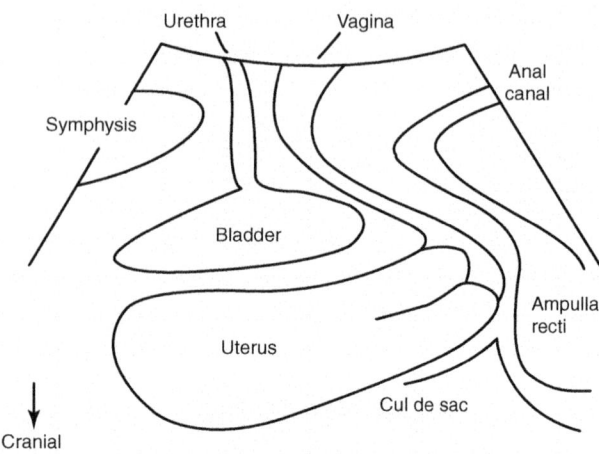

Fig. 4.2 Schema of normal pelvic anatomy by perineal ultrasound

The dynamic examination consists of studying pelvic organs at rest, at Valsalva maneuver, and under levator ani contraction [30–34].

- *Anterior compartment*: ultrasound demonstrates urethral and bladder prolapse during maximum Valsalva maneuver (Fig. 4.3a) but provides supplementary information respect to the physical examination. The study of the angle between the proximal urethra and the trigone, called retrovesical angle, enables to distinguish two different clinical situations: cystocele and cystourethrocele, first described by Green in 1960. Cystocele, defined by isolated bladder prolapse and normal retrovesical angle (90–120°), is associated with voiding dysfunction and seldom with urinary incontinence, while cystourethrocele, with an open retrovesical angle >140°, is characterized by stress urinary incontinence. Comparative studies have mostly shown good correlations between radiologic and ultrasound data.
- *Central compartment*: the study of the central compartment less benefits of ultrasound because in this case clinical examination is precise and exhaustive. Dynamic ultrasound clearly shows the descent of the cervix and supports the study of the relationship between the displaced uterine body and the anterior or posterior vaginal wall to better understand the different clinical manifestations and explaining symptoms of voiding dysfunction or obstructed defecation (Fig. 4.3b).
  In case of hysterectomy, the study of vault descent may be hindered by a concomitant rectocele or enterocele.
- *Posterior compartment*: ultrasound study of the posterior compartment adds important information to the clinical evaluation about the etiology of a posterior colpocele (Fig. 4.4). Different clinical conditions pose the problem of differential diagnosis: it may be related to rectocele, with defect of the rectovaginal septum, to an excessive distensibility without anatomical damage, to enterocele or to a combination of rectocele and enterocele. Rectocele is clearly identified by the herniation of the rectum into the vagina, while in case of enterocele, the hernia contains small bowel or sigmoid colon. The perineal ultrasound enables to

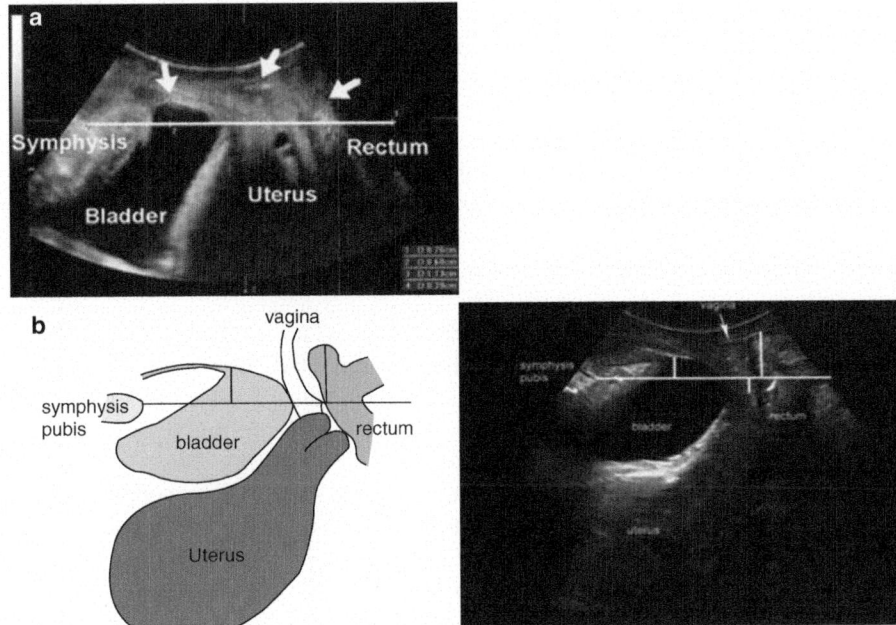

Fig. 4.3 (**a**) Pelvic organ descent as measured by perineal ultrasound. (**b**) Pelvic organ descent as measured with transperineal ultrasound

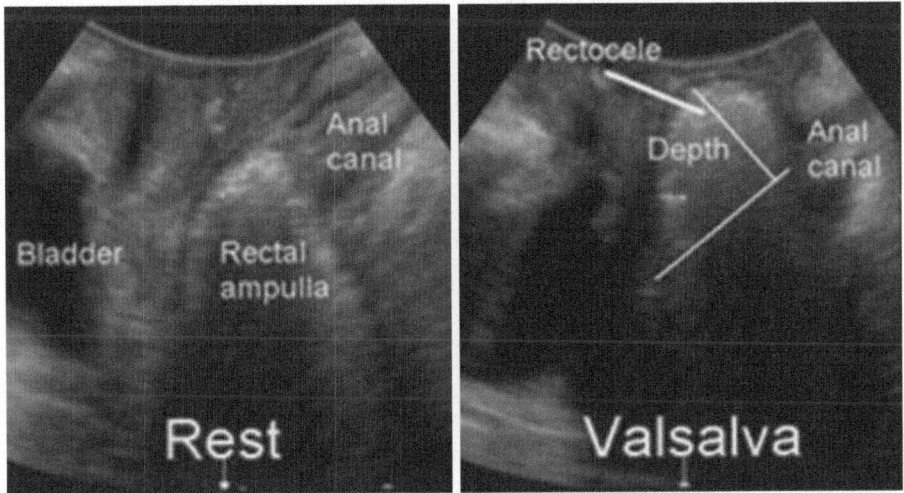

Fig. 4.4 Quantification of rectocele

identify rectal intussusception too, finding the invagination of the rectal wall into the rectal lumen. The possibility to precisely identify the damage, associated with a fairly good correlation with clinical assessment of prolapse, allows the surgeon to decide whether or not to proceed with more invasive endoanal investigations and to determine the best treatment approach. An ultrasound diagnosis of rectocele or rectal intussusception is highly correlated to X-ray imaging findings with the advantage of a high tolerability and greater economy.

Other important parameters related to genital prolapse:

- *Post-voiding residual (PVR) urine*: ultrasound provides a valid estimation of the post-voiding residual urine volume that is particularly important in case of medium high-stage cystocele characterized by voiding dysfunction. The ultrasound bladder volumes can be evaluated using three formulas proposed by Haylen (volume in mL = height × depth × 5.9 − 14.6), Dietz (volume in mL = height × depth × 5.6), and Dicuio (volume in mL = height × depth × transverse × 0.5), and the volumes determined by the three different formulas show strong correlations with the real bladder volume (Fig. 4.5) [35–37].
- *Bladder wall thickness* (BWT): anterior prolapse is the cause of chronic obstruction that can lead to the development of overactive bladder; the measurement of BWT is a useful parameter to evaluate bladder function. An increased medium value is associated to overactive bladder and may be correlated to postoperative de novo urge incontinence. As the bladder distension presses the walls risking to provide altered values, this measurement should be taken at volumes ≤50 mL, though there is still no standardization. The technique consists of taking measures from three sites that are anterior wall, trigone, and dome and calculate an average value (Fig. 4.6) [38].

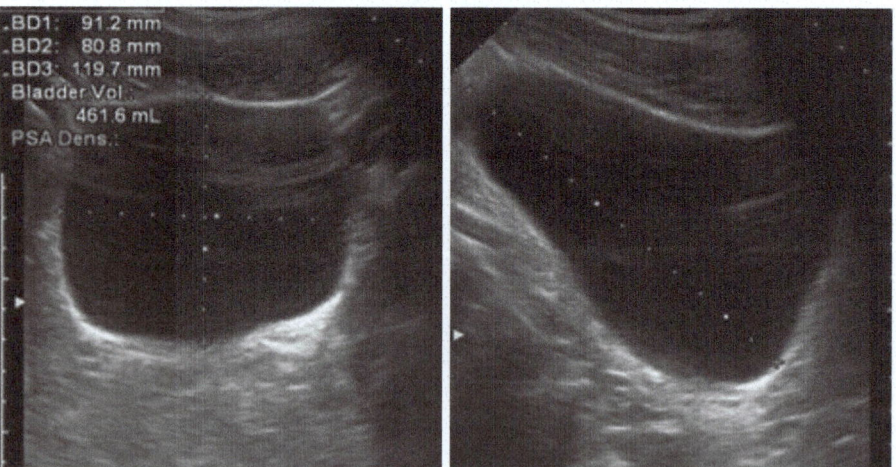

Fig. 4.5 Bladder volume quantification

Fig. 4.6 Measurement of detrusor wall thickness

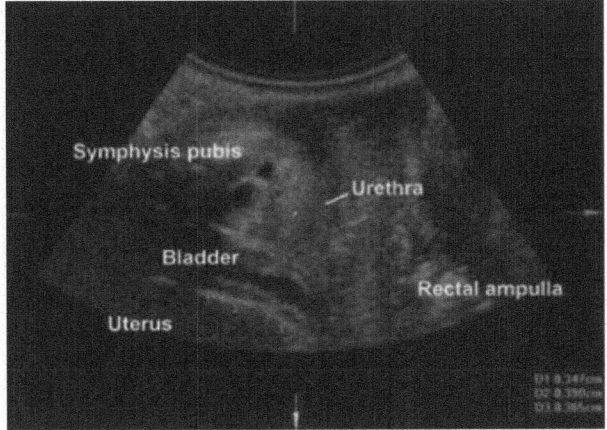

4.5.2   Magnetic Resonance Imaging

Magnetic resonance imaging (MRI) could be useful for more complex cases of genital prolapse, when the physical findings are equivocal or do not explain the patient's symptoms [39].

Advantages of MRI include the lack of ionizing radiation, intrinsic soft tissue contrast capability allowing a detailed visualization of the pelvic floor, and multiplanar imaging. MRI is characterized by increased patient comfort, decreased complexity, and decreased invasiveness compared to radiographic imaging, such as voiding cystourethrography, evacuation proctography, and cystocolpoproctography [40].

Patients may be imaged at rest while straining or while defecating, without contrast material, with vaginal and rectal markers, and with rectal, vaginal, urethral, and bladder contrast material [41, 42]. Imaging may be performed with patients in the supine and upright positions. The dynamic evaluation performed with the patient straining is preferable because prolapse may be visible only with increased abdominal pressure. The variation between resting and straining images helps define the severity of the support defects.

References

1. Lince SL, van Kempen LC, Vierhout ME, et al. A systematic review of clinical studies on hereditary factors in pelvic organ prolapse. Int Urogynecol J. 2012;23(10):1327–36.
2. Kerkhof MH, Hendriks L, Brölmann HA. Changes in connective tissue in patients with pelvic organ prolapse—a review of the currenst literature. Int Urogynecol J Pelvic Floor Dysfunct. 2009;20(4):461–74.
3. Chen HY, Chung YW, Lin WY, et al. Collagen type 3 alpha 1 polymorphism and risk of pelvic organ prolapse. Int J Gynaecol Obstet. 2008;103(1):55–8.
4. Kluivers KB, Dijkstra JR, Hendriks JC, et al. COL3A1 2209G>A is a predictor of pelvic organ prolapse. Int Urogynecol J Pelvic Floor Dysfunct. 2009;20(9):1113–8.

5. Sun MJ, Cheng YS, Sun R, et al. Changes in mitochondrial DNA copy number and extracellular matrix (ECM) proteins in the uterosacral ligaments of premenopausal women with pelvic organ prolapse. Taiwan J Obstet Gynecol. 2016;55(1):9–15.
6. Eser A, Unlubilgin E, Hizli F, et al. Is there a relationship between pelvic organ prolapse and tissue Fibrillin-1 levels? Int Neurourol J. 2015;19(3):164–70.
7. Tetzschner T, Sørensen M, Jønsson L, et al. Delivery and pudendal nerve function. Acta Obstet Gynecol Scand. 1997;76(4):324–31.
8. Alperin M, Cook M, Tuttle LJ, et al. Impact of vaginal parity and aging on the architectural design of pelvic floor muscles. Am J Obstet Gynecol. 2016. [Epub ahead of print];215:312.e1.
9. Novellas S, Chassang M, Verger S, et al. MR features of the levator ani muscle in the immediate postpartum following cesarean delivery. Int Urogynecol J. 2010;21(5):563–8.
10. Laterza RM, Schrutka L, Umek W, et al. Pelvic floor dysfunction after levator trauma 1-year postpartum: a prospective case-control study. Int Urogynecol J. 2015;26(1):41–7.
11. Gyhagen M, Bullarbo M, Nielsen TF, et al. Prevalence and risk factors for pelvic organ prolapse 20 years after childbirth: a national cohort study in singleton primiparae after vaginal or caesarean delivery. BJOG. 2013;120(2):152–60.
12. Glazener C, Elders A, Macarthur C, et al. Childbirth and prolapse: long-term associations with the symptoms and objective measurement of pelvic organ prolapse. BJOG. 2013;120(2):161–8.
13. Marchionni M, Bracco GL, Checcucci V, et al. True incidence of vaginal vault prolapse. Thirteen years of experience. J Reprod Med. 1999;44(8):679–84.
14. Srikrishna S, Robinson D, Cardozo L, et al. Can sex survive pelvic floor surgery? Int Urogynecol J. 2010;21(11):1313–9.
15. Zielinski R, Miller J, Low LK, et al. The relationship between pelvic organ prolapse, genital body image, and sexual health. Neurourol Urodyn. 2012 Sep;31(7):1145–8.
16. Glavind K, Larsen T, Lindquist AS. Sexual function in women before and after surgery for pelvic organ prolapse. Acta Obstet Gynecol Scand. 2015;94(1):80–5.
17. Nichols DH, Randall CL. Vaginal surgery. 4th ed. Baltimore: Williams and Wilkins; 1996.
18. Baden WF, Walker TA. Physical diagnosis in the evaluation of vaginal relaxation. Clin Obstet Gynecol. 1972;15:1055–69.
19. Beecham CT. Classification of vaginal relaxation. Am J Obstet Gynecol. 1980;136(7):957–8.
20. Bump RC, Mattiasson A, Kari B, et al. The standardization of terminology of female pelvic organ prolapse and pelvic floor dysfunction. Am J Obstet Gynecol. 1996;175:10–7.
21. Slieker-ten Hove MC, Pool-Goudzwaard AL, Eijkemans MJ, et al. The prevalence of pelvic organ prolapse symptoms and signs and their relation with bladder and bowel disorders in a general female population. Int Urogynecol J Pelvic Floor Dysfunct. 2009;20(9):1037–45.
22. Haessler AL, Lin LL, Ho MH, et al. Reevaluating occult incontinence. Curr Opin Obstet Gynecol. 2005;17(5):535–40.
23. Reena C, Kekre AN, Kekre N. Occult stress incontinence in women with pelvic organ prolapse. Int J Gynaecol Obstet. 2007;97(1):31–4.
24. Sinha D, Arunkalaivanan AS. Prevalence of occult stress incontinence in continent women with severe genital prolapse. J Obstet Gynaecol. 2007;27(2):174–6.
25. Migliorini GD, Glenning PP. Bonney's test—fact or fiction? Br J Obstet Gynaecol. 1987;94:157–9.
26. Ellström Engh AM, Ekeryd A, Magnusson A, et al. Can de novo stress incontinence after anterior wall repair be predicted? Acta Obstet Gynecol Scand. 2011;90(5):488–93.
27. Bergman A, Koonings PP, Ballard CA. Negative Q-tip test as a risk factor for failed incontinence surgery in women. J Reprod Med. 1989;34(3):193–7.
28. Santoro GA, Wieczorek CI. Pelvic floor disorders. Berlin: Springer; 2010.
29. Santoro GA, Wieczorek CI. Endovaginal ultrasonography: methodology and normal pelvic floor anatomy. Berlin: Springer; 2010.
30. Dietz HP. Ultrasound imaging of the pelvic floor. Part I: two-dimensional aspects. Ultrasound Obstet Gynecol. 2004;23(1):80–92.
31. Dietz HP, Haylen BT, Broome J. Ultrasound in the quantification of female pelvic organ prolapse. Ultrasound Obstet Gynecol. 2001;18(5):511–4.

32. Dietz HP. Why pelvic floor surgeons should utilize ultrasound imaging. Ultrasound Obstet Gynecol. 2006;28(5):629–34.
33. Santoro GA, Wieczorek AP, Dietz HP, et al. State of the art: an integrated approach to pelvic floor ultrasonography. Ultrasound Obstet Gynecol. 2011;37(4):381–96.
34. Tunn R, Petri E. Introital and transvaginal ultrasound as the main tool in the assessment of urogenital and pelvic floor dysfunction: an imaging panel and practical approach. Ultrasound Obstet Gynecol. 2003;22(2):205–13.
35. Haylen BT. Verification of the accuracy and range of transvaginal ultrasound in measuring bladder volumes in women. Br J Urol. 1989;64(4):350–2.
36. Dietz HP, Velez D, Shek KL, et al. Determination of postvoid residual by translabial ultrasound. Int Urogynecol J. 2012;23(12):1749–52.
37. Dicuio M, Pomara G, Menchini Fabris F, et al. Measurements of urinary bladder volume: comparison of five ultrasound calculation methods in volunteers. Arch Ital Urol Androl. 2005;77(1):60–2.
38. Lekskulchai O, Dietz HP. Detrusor wall thickness as a test for detrusor overactivity in women. Ultrasound Obstet Gynecol. 2008;32(4):535–9.
39. Pannu HK, Kaufman HS, Cundiff GW, et al. Dynamic MR imaging of pelvic organ prolapse: spectrum of abnormalities. Radiographics. 2000;20(6):1567–82.
40. Kaufman HS, Buller JL, Thompson JR, et al. Dynamic pelvic magnetic resonance imaging and cystocolpoproctography alter surgical management of pelvic floor disorders. Dis Colon Rectum. 2001;44:1575–83. discussion 1583-1584.
41. Yang A, Mostwin JL, Rosenshein NB, et al. Pelvic floor descent in women: dynamic evaluation with fast MR imaging and cinematic display. Radiology. 1991;179:25–33.
42. Lienemann A, Anthuber C, Baron A, et al. Dynamic MR colpocystorectography assessing pelvic floor descent. Eur Radiol. 1997;7:1309–17.

Urodynamic Prolapse Assessment: When and Why

5

Andrea Braga, Martina Milanesi, and Giulio Del Popolo

5.1 Introduction

The role of urodynamic studies (UDS) before prolapse surgery is controversial and remains one of the most debated issues in urogynaecology [1]. POP and lower urinary tract symptoms (LUTS) often coexist as they may have a similar underlying pathophysiology. Up to 96% of women with POP report LUTS with mixed urinary incontinence predominating [1]. Nevertheless, it has not been possible to reach a universal consensus on the role of UDS before prolapse surgery, especially in women with concomitant symptomatic or occult stress urinary incontinence (SUI). The implementation of powerful and sophisticated instruments, such as artificial neural networks or multiple linear regression, does not permit an accurate diagnosis of the lower urinary tract dysfunction based on symptoms and pelvic examination findings [2]. The data on the use of UDS in patients with uncomplicated and pure SUI are conflicting and heterogeneous [3, 4]. Very few data exist on the role of UDS in the preoperative evaluation of women with POP. The latest recommendations of the International Consultation on Incontinence for the management of POP suggest only selective use of UDS when the results would alter the planned treatment [5]. It is clear that UDS could add some information in women undergoing pelvic organ prolapse surgery and could facilitate counselling of patients. However, there is no evidence that the outcome of surgery is altered by prior UDS. The question is whether how UDS can really change the choice of surgery and its outcome in women with POP (Fig. 5.1).

A. Braga
Department of Obstetrics and Gynecology, EOC—Beata Vergine Hospital, Mendrisio, Switzerland

M. Milanesi
Department of Urology, Careggi University Hospital, Florence, Italy

G. Del Popolo (✉)
Department of Neuro-Urology, Careggi University Hospital, Florence, Italy
e-mail: delpopolog@aou-careggi.toscana.it

© Springer International Publishing AG, part of Springer Nature 2018   61
V. Li Marzi, M. Serati (eds.), *Management of Pelvic Organ Prolapse*,
Urodynamics, Neurourology and Pelvic Floor Dysfunctions,
https://doi.org/10.1007/978-3-319-59195-7_5

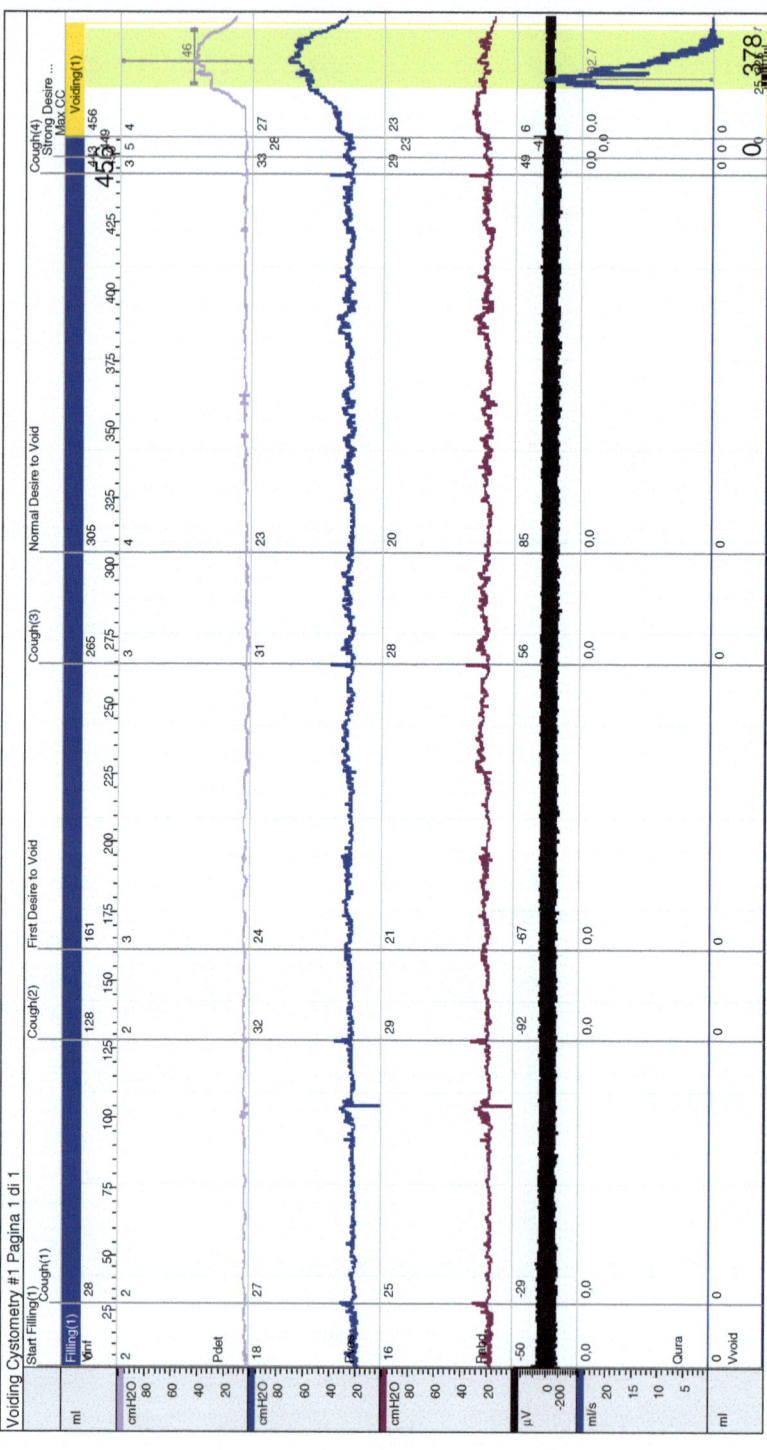

Fig. 5.1 UDS with no reduction of POP presurgery: BOO pattern at P/F study

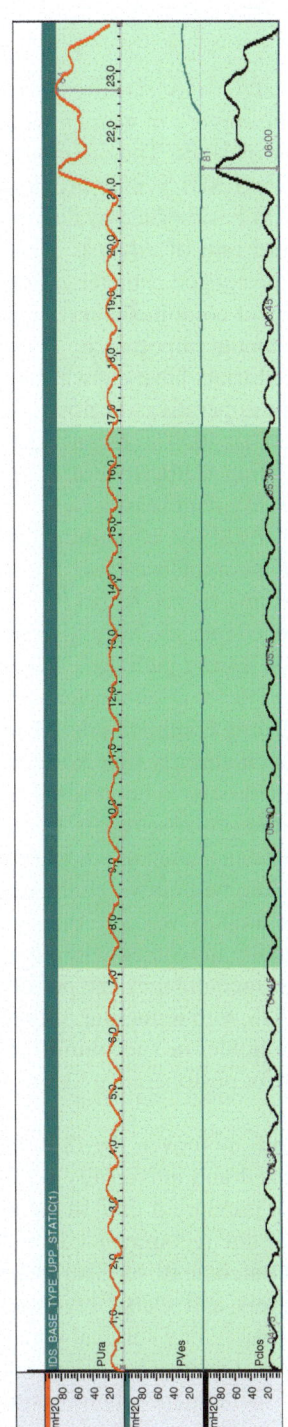

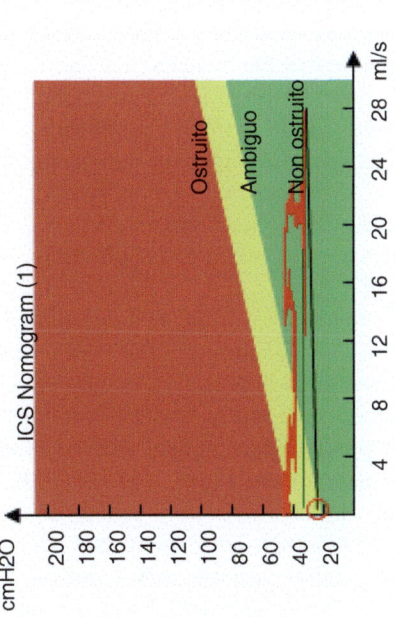

Fig. 5.1 (continued)

5.1.1 POP and Stress Urinary Incontinence

In 2000, Weber and Walters developed decision-analytic models to evaluate the cost-effectiveness of basic office evaluation before the surgery in women with prolapse and SUI symptoms and contrasted it with that of UDS. They demonstrated that UDS before surgery in women with prolapse and SUI symptoms does not improve cure rates and is not cost-effective relative to basic office evaluation [6]. Combination surgery is associated with an increased rate of adverse events [7] (major bleeding complications, bladder perforation, prolonged catheterization, urinary tract infections) and higher cost. As the benefits of combined surgery should outweigh its risks, careful patient selection is of paramount importance.

A number of well-designed randomized controlled trials have shown that concomitant continence surgery reduces the risk of postoperative de novo SUI in women without SUI who are undergoing POP surgery [8, 9]. The recent outcomes following vaginal prolapse repair and midurethral sling (OPUS) trial compared anterior vaginal prolapse repair with or without a concomitant tension-free vaginal tape (TVT) sling procedure in stress-continent women [8]. At 12 months, urinary incontinence (allowing for subsequent treatment of incontinence) was present in 27.3% and 43.0% of patients in the sling and sham groups, respectively ($P = 0.002$). It is important to underline that the de novo incontinence rate was very high in both groups, although only women without symptoms of SUI were included. The rate of bladder perforation was higher in the sling group (6.7% vs. 0%), as were rates of urinary tract infection (31.0% vs. 18.3%), major bleeding complications (3.1% vs. 0%) and VD (3.7% vs. 0%). The authors estimated that in this asymptomatic female population, at 12 months, 6.3 prophylactic slings would have to be inserted to prevent one woman from becoming stress incontinent after prolapse repair. In conclusion, the authors stated that if SUI has been documented in a woman preoperatively, then it is possible that the benefits of a concomitant sling will outweigh the risks; if not, the risk-benefit ratio is less predictable [8]. The authors who are in favour of UDS in women with POP often claim that this evaluation in women without symptoms of SUI enables the demonstration of occult stress incontinence and possibly its treatment. Furthermore, they support preoperative UDS with reduction of prolapse (semi-reclined position with gauze a pessary, sponge holder or speculum) because several studies have shown negative predictive values for postoperative SUI of more than 90% [10].

However, this has not been well-demonstrated and, moreover, the best way to unmask the occult SUI during UDS is not standardized and universally accepted. The use of abdominal leak point pressure and urethral pressure profile in the evaluation of women with stress urinary incontinence is not recommended by AUA guidelines to predict which patient will have the best outcome of surgical treatment for stress urinary incontinence [11]. In 2007, Roovers and Oelke reviewed the impact of UDS in the diagnostic workup of patients undergoing surgical correction of genital prolapse [12]. They stated that occult SUI is diagnosed in about 50% of patients with genital prolapse not reporting stress incontinence before surgery. However, the authors underlined that it is unknown which barrier test is preferred to assess the presence of occult urodynamic stress incontinence. In addition, it is unknown whether occult SUI can be equally effectively diagnosed by non-urodynamic tests such as a pessary test or a Sims' speculum. Roovers and Oelke also found that the combination of prolapse and stress incontinence surgery not only has the advantage of attempting to solve two problems at the same time but also carries an increased risk of unwanted side effects, of which VD and DO are the most important [12].

The most recent randomized trial on this topic enrolled 80 patients with POP and occult SUI who were randomly assigned to prolapse surgery alone without a sling or prolapse surgery with concurrent TVT. After 24 months, the authors observed similar subjective and objective outcomes in the two groups, and they concluded that these results support a policy that routine insertion of a sling in women with occult SUI at the time of prolapse repair is questionable and should be subject to shared decision-making between clinician and patient [13]. Regarding the type of continence surgery, we could use guidance from studies comparing different midurethral tapes without excluding concomitant POP surgery. A retropubic tape appears to be more suitable than a transobturator tape in women with intrinsic sphincter deficiency, diagnosed using urethral pressure profilometry and/or Valsalva leak point pressures [14]. As the placement of the retropubic tape is closer to perpendicular to the urethral axis, it creates greater circumferential compression of the urethra and provides better support.

A recently publish systematic review included seven randomized trials to evaluate prolapse surgery with or without incontinence surgery in women with POP [7]. The authors considered studies that included women without urinary symptoms and studies that included women with occult SUI. Interestingly, this meta-analysis showed that in asymptomatic women, combination surgery resulted in a lower incidence of de novo subjective SUI and the need for subsequent anti-incontinence surgery; however, the rates of de novo objective SUI were similar in the group of women undergoing incontinence surgery and the group without anti-incontinence surgery. In the subgroup of women with occult SUI, there was a lower incidence of objective SUI after combination surgery but with a higher rate of adverse events and a higher rate of prolonged catheterization. It seems evident that even if UDS could diagnose occult SUI using validated and standardized methods (which is not the case at this time), there would be no scientific evidence that it is always appropriate and convenient to associate the two surgical procedures. Therefore, the UDS diagnosis would still not be able to change with absolute certainty the surgical choice.

5.1.2 POP and Urgency/Urgency Incontinence/Voiding Dysfunctions

UDS may also identify patients at risk of persistence or development of postoperative urgency/urgency incontinence and voiding dysfunctions (VD). A significantly reduced cure rate with antimuscarinics in women with OAB and concomitant anterior vaginal wall descent has been demonstrated [15]. These symptoms are associated with poor patient satisfaction as the majority of the patients expect complete postoperative resolution of all their LUTS. The presence of preoperative DO [16] has been identified as a predictive factor for persistent urgency and urgency incontinence after POP surgery, although Nguyen et al. found that in approximately two thirds of women with POP and concomitant symptomatic DO, there is resolution of DO after prolapse repair [17]. Other recognized predictive factors are higher voiding pressure at maximal flow (PdetQmax) [18] and higher bladder outlet obstruction index, calculated as PdetQmax—2Qmax [19, 20]. Thus, urodynamic information can facilitate tailored counselling of patients regarding the need for postoperative treatment for urgency/urgency incontinence such as antimuscarinic agents. Preoperative poor detrusor contractility is associated with postoperative VD [16]. Identifying patients likely to develop postoperative VD may be useful in helping to accurately shape patient expectations and identify those most likely to benefit from preoperative teaching of clean intermittent self-catheterization (CISC) or insertion of a suprapubic catheter at the time of surgery if they cannot perform CISC.

Conclusions

UDS are a series of objective tests which improve our understanding of urinary dysfunctions and their interaction with POP, such as a preoperative DO or a occult SUI, but this information rarely leads to a change in the management plan or the type of surgical procedure. Moreover, surgical correction of prolapse can improve not only the symptom of vaginal bulging but also the symptoms of OAB and could cure the concomitant SUI. As a matter of fact, the surgical procedure is not only aimed to remodel anatomy but also to improve or maintain pelvic floor functions, including bowel, bladder and sexual activity. However, UDS offer valuable information to the surgeon that could potentially improve decision-making and overall patient management. Urodynamic data could also help patients accurately assess the risks and benefits of surgery and facilitate optimal preoperative counselling directed towards appropriate patient expectations as well as guide proactive management of postoperative symptoms. Thus, urodynamic knowledge is of utmost fundamental for the urogynecologist surgeon.

Nevertheless, new well-designed randomized studies are necessary to improve our understanding of this topic.

References

1. Serati M, Giarenis I, Meschia M, Cardozo L. Role of urodynamics before prolapse surgery. Int Urogynecol J. 2015;26:165–8.
2. Serati M, Salvatore S, Siesto G, Cattoni E, Braga A, Sorice P, et al. Urinary symptoms and urodynamic findings in women with pelvic organ prolapse: is there a correlation? Results of an artificial neural network analysis. Eur Urol. 2011;60:253–60.

3. Weber AM, Taylor RJ, Wei JT, Lemack G, Piedmonte MR, Walters MD. The cost-effectiveness of preoperative testing (basic office assessment vs. urodynamics) for stress urinary incontinence in women. BJU Int. 2002;89:356–63.
4. Digesu GA, Hendricken C, Fernando R, Khullar V. Do women with pure stress urinary incontinence need urodynamics? Rology. 2009;74:278–81.
5. Abrams P, Andersson KE, Apostolidis A, et al. Recommendation of the International Scientific Committee: evaluation and treatment of urinary incontinence, pelvic organ prolapse and faecal incontinence. In: Abrams P, Cardozo L, Wagg A, Wein A, editors. Incontinence: 6th International Consultation on Incontinence. Tokyo: ICUD-ICS; 2016. p. 2549–97.
6. Weber AM, Walters MD. Cost-effectiveness of urodynamic testing before surgery for women with pelvic organ prolapse and stress urinary incontinence. Am J Obstet Gynecol. 2000;183:1338–47.
7. van der Ploeg J, van der Steen A, Oude Rengerink K, van der Vaart C, Roovers J. Prolapse surgery with or without stress incontinence surgery for pelvic organ prolapse: a systematic review and meta-analysis of randomised trials. BJOG. 2014;121:537–47.
8. Wei JT, Nygaard I, Richter HE, Nager CW, Barber MD, Kenton K, et al. A midurethral sling to reduce incontinence after vaginal prolapse repair. N Engl J Med. 2012;366:2358–67.
9. Brubaker L, Nygaard I, Richter HE, Visco A, Weber AM, Cundiff GW, et al. Two-year outcomes after sacrocolpopexy with and without burch to prevent stress urinary incontinence. Obstet Gynecol. 2008;112:49–55.
10. Srikrishna S, Robinson D, Cardozo L. Ringing the changes in evaluation of urogenital prolapse. Int Urogynecol J. 2011;22:171–5.
11. Christian Winters J, Dmochowski RR, Goldman HB, Anthony Herndon CD, Kobashi KC, Kraus SR, Lemack GE, Nitti VW, Rovner ES, Wein AJ. Urodynamic studies in adults: AUA/SUFU Guideline. J Urol. 2012. https://doi.org/10.1016/j.juro.2012.09.081.
12. Roovers JP, Oelke M. Clinical relevance of urodynamic investigation tests prior to surgical correction of genital prolapse: a literature review. Int Urogynecol J. 2007;18:455–60.
13. Schierlitz L, Dwyer PL, Rosamilia A, et al. Pelvic organ prolapse surgery with and without tension-free vaginal tape in women with occult or asymptomatic urodynamic stress incontinence: a randomised controlled trial. Int Urogynecol J. 2014;25:33–40.
14. Schierlitz L, Dwyer PL, Rosamilia A, Murray C, Thomas E, De Souza A, et al. Three year follow-up of tension-free vaginal tape compared with transobturator tape in women with stress urinary incontinence and intrinsic sphincter deficiency. Obstet Gynecol. 2012;119:321–7.
15. Salvatore S, Serati M, Ghezzi F, Uccella S, Cromi A, Bolis P. Efficacy of tolterodine in women with detrusor overactivity and anterior vaginal wall prolapse: is it the same? BJOG. 2007;114:1436–8.
16. Araki I, Haneda Y, Mikami Y, Takeda M. Incontinence and detrusor dysfunction associated with pelvic organ prolapse: clinical value of preoperative urodynamic evaluation. Int Urogynecol J Pelvic Floor Dysfunct. 2009;20:1301–6.
17. Nguyen JK, Bahatia NN. Resolution of motor urge incontinence after surgical repair of pelvic organ prolapse. J Urol. 2001;166:2263–6.
18. Fletcher SG, Haverkorn RM, Yan J, Lee JJ, Zimmern PE, Lemack GE. Demographic and urodynamic factors associated with persistent OAB after anterior compartment prolapse repair. Neurourol Urodyn. 2010;29:1414–8.
19. Lee DM, Ryu YW, Lee YT, Ahn SH, Han JH, Yum SH. A predictive factor in overactive bladder symptoms improvement after combined anterior vaginal wall prolapse repair: a pilot study. Korean J Urol. 2012;53:405–9.
20. Abdullah B, Nomura J, Moriyama S, Huang T, Tokiwa S, Togo M. Clinical and urodynamic assessment in patients with pelvic organ prolapse before and after laparoscopic sacrocolpopexy. Int Urogynecol J. 2017;28(10):543–1549. [Epub ahead of print].

Part III

Treatment Options

Pelvic Floor Muscle Training and Prolapse: Prevention or Treatment?

Antonella Biroli and Gian Franco Lamberti

Pelvic organ prolapse (POP), the descent of the pelvic organs due to deficiencies in the pelvic support system, is a very common problem. Up to 40% of women aged 45–85 years have at least stage II POP according to POP-Q staging [1], even though only 10–20% of them seek medical care [2]. Pelvic floor muscle training has been proposed for its prevention and treatment.

POP may be asymptomatic, especially when the descending organs are above the hymen. Feeling of heaviness or pressure in the vagina is the most specific symptom of genital prolapse, followed by voiding and bowel difficulties. The prevalence of symptomatic prolapse (feeling or seeing a vaginal bulge) is reported to be about 3–12% [3].

Urinary incontinence can coexist, but its relationship with prolapse is still under discussion. Actually, although POP and stress urinary incontinence (SUI) share some common risk factors, some differences may exist: a family history seems to be a stronger risk factor for SUI, while an older age for POP; obesity seems to be a stronger risk factor for SUI, while parity, higher foetal weight, and forceps are more related to POP [2].

Surgery is a valid option for POP treatment since it is effective in correcting anatomical abnormalities, but recurrence is possible, and persisting or "de novo" pelvic floor symptoms can decrease patient satisfaction after surgery.

Pelvic floor muscle training (PFMT) increases pelvic floor muscle strength and function, so it may help to prevent prolapse worsening and improve specific prolapse symptoms, as feeling of vaginal bulging or heaviness, and other associated symptoms, as urinary and anal incontinence, too.

A. Biroli (✉)
Neurologic and Autonomic Dysfunctions Rehabilitation Center, Physical Medicine and Rehabilitation Unit, San Giovanni Bosco Hospital, Torino, Italia
e-mail: biran@virgilio.it

G. F. Lamberti
Department of Medicina Riabilitativa Ospedaliera di Fossano dell'ASL CN1,
ASL CN1, Cuneo, Italy

© Springer International Publishing AG, part of Springer Nature 2018
V. Li Marzi, M. Serati (eds.), *Management of Pelvic Organ Prolapse*,
Urodynamics, Neurourology and Pelvic Floor Dysfunctions,
https://doi.org/10.1007/978-3-319-59195-7_6

PFMT may be considered a first-line therapy, especially when the prolapse is mild. Moreover, in the last decade, PFMT was proposed to augment the effect of surgery in women with pelvic organ prolapse, even though, currently, there is insufficient evidence to support adding perioperative PFMT to surgery [4, 5].

PFMT can virtually be offered to all patients with POP, as no adverse effect was seen. Patients with advanced prolapse, that unlikely can resolve their problem with PFMT, also may have beneficial effects on symptoms.

6.1   Prolapse and Rehabilitation: Theoretical Basis

Women with prolapse generate less vaginal closure force during a maximal contraction of pelvic floor muscles than controls [6]. Prolapse is associated with reduced PFM strength in the postpartum period too [7]. Pelvic floor muscle training increases PFM strength, so it represents a good option in the management of pelvic organ prolapse [8], but the real mechanism that underlies its effect is unknown.

Two main hypotheses about its mode of action involve [9]:

– Improvement of the structural support of the pelvis, resulting in a higher location of the levator plate and of the pelvic organs, in a narrowing of the pelvic openings and an increase of PFM tone and strength.
– Prevention of pelvic organ descent during cough or other physical exertion by intentional contraction of the PFM, before and during the increase in abdominal pressure.

These two different hypotheses imply two different treatment approaches.

To achieve better pelvic support, as stated by the first hypothesis, the rehabilitative treatment should apply strength training principles. Training should involve at least three sets of 8–12 close to maximum contraction 2–4 days a week [9].

On the other hand, to contrast the pelvic organ descent during increases in abdominal pressure by contracting pelvic floor muscles, as stated by the second hypothesis, it is necessary to teach this voluntary contraction to the patients. This type of pelvic floor muscle contraction was named "the knack" [10]. Associating PFM activity to different movements that increase abdominal pressure (as cough, sneezing, clearing the throat, physical exertions) may subsequently reinforce pelvic muscles by repeated contractions. Moreover, after numerous repetitions, this voluntary manoeuvre to contrast pelvic organ descent may shift to an automatic movement (coordination training).

Exercises for strength training and knack learning can both be used during rehabilitation sessions.

Unfortunately, there is a lack of evidence about the optimal PFMT regimen for prolapse prevention or treatment. This is not surprising, if considering that PFMT was initially proposed for the treatment of female urinary incontinence (level A evidence exists that it is effective) [11], and in spite of the great number of studies and the time passed since the acknowledgement of its effectiveness, a standard protocol for PFMT is not yet available. The optimal number of contraction repetitions, daily training frequency, timing and duration of contractions type of exercise are still under discussion [12]. PFMT was used for the treatment of pelvic organ prolapse in more recent years, and, similarly, the training protocols vary widely.

Usually, strength training implies instructions about correct PFM contraction, avoiding apnea and recruitment of accessory muscles. Attention should be paid to obtain not only a vaginal closure movement but an inward-lift movement too. Exercises for both tonic and phasic PFM activity may be proposed, to improve the tonic pelvic support, on one side, and the phasic contraction needed to counteract abdominal pressure during cough and physical exertion, on the other side. PFM exercises should be performed in different conditions, from lying to an upright position. Training can increase strength, power and endurance of pelvic floor muscles and drive to neuromuscular facilitation. It was demonstrated in women that, after brief training, voluntary pelvic floor contraction elevates the bladder neck and, after intensive training, bladder neck is elevated in functional conditions and also at rest [10, 13]. Additionally, pelvic floor muscle training can close the levator hiatus and elevate the resting position of bladder and rectum [14].

Some authors applied biofeedback therapy or electrical stimulation if PFM was weak (grade 0 or 1 on modified Oxford grading system) [15], although there is no available evidence to support such an approach.

Prolapse prevention and treatment is founded on pelvic floor muscle treatment, that is the only evidence-based rehabilitation modality. Nevertheless, pelvic organ position depends on the balance of opposite forces. Gravitational force and abdominal pressure, that increases in standing position and during efforts, are responsible for the descent of pelvic organs, while fascia and ligaments have a "pull up" and pelvic floor muscles a "push up" effect on viscera. From this point of view, an important unanswered question is if an intervention to reduce downward forces is feasible and useful too.

Rib cage mobility-oriented breathing exercises in association with pelvic floor contraction, aimed to reduce downward pressure on viscera, have been proposed [16]. Preliminary studies showed more thoracic kyphosis in women affected by POP and hypothesised that a change in respiratory dynamics and the consequent increase of abdominal pressure were responsible for that [17, 18]. On these bases, if data were confirmed, an intervention to correct postural kyphosis and rib cage closure, if present, may be reasonable, when added to PFMT.

Some studies have well described the different patterns of movement that can be used to cough, as well as to do efforts [19]. Actually, coughing, sneezing and blowing the nose are the result of a forced expiration obtained by contracting mainly the intercostal muscles and diaphragm or, as an alternative, lower transversus abdominis, oblique, and pelvic floor muscles. These two different patterns of movement generate the same final effect, e.g. a cough, as the result of differently oriented forces. Pelvic organs also are subjected to forces that create the intrathoracic pressure increase needed to cough, but how much all of these results in a "push out" effect depends on the pattern of movement. So, teaching a woman how to cough and to do efforts may be very important when preventing and treating prolapse [20], even if today there is no availability of studies to support it.

6.2 Prolapse Assessment: A Rehabilitative Point of View

Prolapse is a dynamic condition. Anatomical and functional damages are responsible for it, but its expression is variable, as it changes in different positions and conditions. Fatigue associated with prolonged standing accounts for worsening of bulging and pressure vaginal symptoms in the evening; on the contrary nocturnal rest is associated with a lesser bulging in the morning.

Prolapse evaluation is usually performed with the patient straining so that maximum descent is attained. The adoption of a standardised quantification, as the pelvic organ prolapse quantification (POP-Q) or its simplified version [21] is recommended. The maximum descent during straining is measured and used to define the prolapse stage (0–4). So prolapse stage during maximal straining is commonly used to describe prolapse.

From a rehabilitative point of view, such an evaluation is incomplete. Actually, during a correct straining effort (that is not synonymous with Valsalva manoeuvre), the pelvic floor should be relaxed. The patient is asked to push out her prolapse, so only the passive elements of the support system are evaluable. Rehabilitation acts especially on active elements of the support system, fundamentally the pelvic floor muscles, which in this way are not well functionally evaluated. On the other side, the assessment of pelvic floor muscle strength, using a validated system as the modified Oxford grading system, is essential but insufficient to describe the effect of the PFM contraction on pelvic organ position.

Finally, prolapse staging is insufficient to describe prolapse expression during common life (How much is the feeling of prolapse descent present over the course of the day? Is the woman able to partially reposition pelvic organs using pelvic floor contraction or reducing abdominal pressure?) that is an important goal for rehabilitation. Prolapse-specific questionnaires, like P-QOL [22] and patient-oriented measures, help to assess patients affected by prolapse more than prolapse by itself.

Prolapse assessment may be completed by evaluating prolapse behaviour under different conditions in sequence [23]:

- During straining, as traditionally, making sure that the woman pushes correctly down the viscera (some patients are not able to relax the pelvic floor and show incoordination during straining).
- After straining, evaluating the presence and amount of a spontaneous inward return movement of the prolapse. Prolapses, although similar during straining, show different behaviours when straining is given up. Some prolapses return quickly to an upper position, and others remain in a descended one, with little change despite the end of straining. The reason for this different response is not clear, but a return movement may be interpreted as the sign of residual effectiveness and elasticity of the passive elements contributing to pelvic support.

– During pelvic floor contraction, evaluating its effect on prolapse. Little or absent effect may be due to different conditions, such as weak pelvic floor or pelvic floor's inability to act on pelvic organ descent too. The effect of pelvic floor contraction on prolapse can be seen by clinical examination, ultrasound and MRI.

6.3   Evidence in Rehabilitation for POP

Conservative treatments to improve the function of pelvic floor muscles (PFM) and support, such as pelvic floor muscle training (PFMT), vaginal pessaries and lifestyle intervention (avoiding of lifting and weight loss), are often recommended [24, 25].

Women with POP have reduced PFM strength [6, 26–28], and the severity of POP seems to increase with increasing PFM dysfunction [29, 30]; studies indicated that PFMT could effectively support—improving strength, endurance and coordination—the pelvic organs in the normal anatomic position by contracting pelvic floor muscles before and during any increase in abdominal pressure [25, 31].

In addition, structural support of pelvic floor muscles is significantly improved by performing PFMT [32]. Pelvic floor muscle training has no adverse effects, and anatomic understanding of PFM function provides a theoretical basis for strength training of the PFM to be effective in prevention and treatment of POP [9].

Various studies have been published on the effectiveness of rehabilitation exercises in the treatment of prolapse; some are pilot studies of quite small populations or whose conclusions may be affected by methodological limitations [33–38].

With these reservations, the exercises have proven to be effective in mitigating anatomical damage to the anterior and posterior vaginal walls, reducing symptomatology in POP of grade 1 or 2 and improving sexual function in women affected by POP, with improved perceived quality of life and results persisting for up to 2 years after the treatment ends. According to some authors, the benefits gained from PFMT compared with a "watchful waiting" approach, while present, are not at a clinically relevant level [39].

When comparing PFMT plus the provision of a self-instruction manual with the manual alone, PFMT group showed greater improvement in POP symptoms [40].

A trial [33] describes the treatment associated with PFMT and dietary suggestions (plenty of fluids and vegetables to avoid constipation and the resulting need to "push" when defecating), compared with no treatment in a population of 654 women aged >60 years; a worsening grade of prolapse was observed mainly in women who received no treatment.

Broadly speaking, the RCTs presented in the literature compare PFMT combined with behavioural changes in everyday life with behavioural changes alone.

All the studies of this type highlight an improvement in symptomatology in favour of PFMT combined with behavioural changes; the latter generally involves performing a manoeuvre, whereby the pelvi-perineal muscles are contracted in anticipation of an increase in intra-abdominal pressure (the "knack"), together with advice not to push during defecation [41, 42] and general lifestyle advice (reducing heavy activities and weight loss) [41, 43–45].

Unfortunately, no data are available comparing behavioural changes alone with nontreatment; thus we have no data on the effectiveness of lifestyle changes alone.

Large-scale clinical trials have confirmed the improvement in subjective symptomatology and positive anatomical changes resulting from the exercises [40, 46], albeit without precisely analysing the influence of any other conservative treatments but describing a more favourable outcome at 24 months compared with "wait and see" [47].

The importance of possible different effectiveness of the exercises on prolapses of different types and grades, as well as a possible positive influence of the spontaneous clinical evolution of the prolapse itself, is emphasised by a recent clinical trial that confirms the benefits of the exercises at 12 months. The reduction in subjective symptomatology represents the primary outcome of the clinical trial; this is the principal objective that motivates a person to begin the rehabilitation process and a fact that does not necessarily correlate with the anatomical improvement of the prolapse. On the other hand, not all women who perform the therapeutic exercises improve, and the authors hypothesise that, to optimise their effectiveness, the criteria for rehabilitative training must be further defined [48].

PFMT effectiveness is confirmed by a meta-analysis that expresses the hypothesis that improvement in symptoms and grade of prolapse may be possible by increasing muscle strength and endurance through intensive exercises practised over a long period [49].

To date, there is no specific scientific evidence in the literature relating to the effectiveness of PFMT for the primary prevention of prolapse or when it occurs.

There are conflicting data regarding the benefits of the prevention and treatment of POP in primiparous women. A recent RCT reported no significant risk difference in POP or bladder neck position between PFMT group and control group in primiparous women following vaginal delivery [50]. Another study reported that the prevalence of prolapse symptoms or objectively measured POP did not differ at 12 years between PFMT (instruction on three occasions) and control group [51].

Considering that surgical management of POP is frequent, it is extremely interesting to examine data about the relationship between PFMT and prolapse surgery.

A prospective, non-randomised study [52] suggests that among women affected by POP, the perceived improvement is greater in the group having undergone surgery than in the group treated with conservative techniques.

Data available in the literature seem to indicate that PFMT combined or not with behavioural treatment does not improve the result of surgical treatment [15, 53, 54]. A study showing positive results by PFMT underlies that findings need to be confirmed by broader trials [55].

Finally, a previous Cochrane systematic review [56] demonstrated that PFMT as a treatment for women with POP resulted "in a significant improvement of prolapse symptoms and severity of POP", but "reliable evidence from high-quality randomized trials was necessary"; the recently updated literature search of randomised controlled trials [8] confirmed that PFMT might improve symptoms and reduce the severity of prolapse (level of evidence, 1; grade of recommendation, A).

References

1. Slieker-ten Hove MC, Pool-Goudzwaard AL, Eijkemans MJ, et al. The prevalence of pelvic organ prolapse symptoms and signs and their relation with bladder and bowel disorders in a general female population. Int Urogynecol J Pelvic Floor Dysfunct. 2009;20(9):1037–45.
2. Rodriguez-Mias N, Martinez-Franco E, Aguado J, et al. Pelvic organ prolapse and stress urinary incontinence, do they share the same risk factors? Eur J Obstet Gynecol Reprod Biol. 2015;190:52–7.
3. Nygaard I, Barber MD, Burgio KL, et al. Prevalence of symptomatic pelvic floor disorders in US women. JAMA. 2008;300(11):1311–6.
4. Zhang FW, Wei F, Wang HL, et al. Does pelvic floor muscle training augment the effect of surgery in women with pelvic organ prolapsed? A systematic review of randomized controlled trials. Neurourol Urodyn. 2016;35(6):666–74.
5. Lakeman MM, Koops SE, Berghmans BC, et al. Peri-operative physiotherapy to prevent recurrent symptoms and treatment following prolapsed surgery: supported by evidence or not? Int Urogynecol J. 2013;24(3):371–5.
6. De Lancey JO, Morgan D, Fenner DE, et al. Comparison of levator ani muscle defects and function in women with and without pelvic organ prolapsed. Obstet Gynecol. 2007;109:295–302.
7. Diez-Itza I, Arrue M, Ibanez L, et al. Postpartum impairment of pelvic floor muscle function: factors involved and association with prolapsed. Int Urogynecol J. 2011;22:1505–11.
8. Dumoulin C, Hunter KF, Moore K, et al. Conservative management for female urinary incontinence and pelvic organ prolapse review 2013: Summary of the 5th International Consultation on Incontinence. Neurourol Urodyn. 2016;35(1):15–20.
9. Bo K. Can pelvic floor muscle training prevent and treat pelvic organ prolapsed? Acta Obstet Gynecol Scand. 2006;85(3):263–8.
10. Miller JM, Perucchini D, Carchidi LT, et al. Pelvic floor muscle contraction during a cough and decreased vesical neck mobility. Obstet Gynecol. 2001;97(2):255–60.
11. Moore K, Domoulin C, Bradley C, et al. Adult conservative management. In: Abrams P, Cardozo L, Khouri AE, Wein A, editors. International consultation on urinary incontinence. 5th ed. Plymbridge: Health Publications Ltd; 2013. p. 1101–95.
12. Hay-Smith J, Herderschee R, Dumoulin C, et al. Comparisons of approaches to pelvic floor muscle training for urinary incontinence in women: an abridged Cochrane systematic review. Eur J Phys Rehabil Med. 2012;48(4):689–705.
13. Balmforth JR, Mantle J, Bidmead J, et al. A prospective observational trial of pelvic floor muscle training for female stress urinary incontinence. BJU Int. 2006;98(4):811–7.
14. Braekken IH, Majida M, Engh ME, et al. Can pelvic floor muscle training reverse pelvic organ prolapse and reduce prolapsed symptoms? An assessor-blinded, randomized, controlled trial. Am J Obstet Gynecol. 2010;203:170e1–7.
15. Frawley HC, Phyllips BA, Bo K, et al. Physiotherapy as an adjunct to prolapsed surgery: an assessor-blinded randomized controlled trial. Neurourol Urodyn. 2010;29:719–25.
16. Calais-Germain B. Le périnée feminine et l'accouchement. Désiris ed. Paris; 2000.
17. Lind LR, Lucente V, Kohn N. Thoracic kyphosis and the prevalence of advanced uterine prolapse. Obstet Gynecol. 1996;87(4):605–9.
18. Nguyen J, Lind R, Choe J, McKindesy F, et al. Lumbosacral spine and pelvic inlet changes associated with pelvic organ prolapsed. Obstet Gynecol. 2000;95:332–6.
19. Sapsford R. Rehabilitation of pelvic floor muscles utilizing trunk stabilization. Man Ther. 2004;9(1):3–12.
20. De Gasquet B. Abdominaux: arretez le massacre. Marabout ed. Paris, 2005.
21. Bump RC, Mattiasson A, Bo K, et al. The standardization of terminology of female pelvic organ prolapse and pelvic floor dysfunction. Am J Obstet Gynecol. 1996;175(1):10–7.
22. Di Gesu GA, Khullar V, Cardozo L, et al. P-QOL: a validated questionnaire to assess the symptoms and quality of life of women with urogenital prolapse. Int Urogynecol J Pelvic Floor Dysfunct. 2005;16(3):176–81.

23. Biroli A. Prolasso genitale e riabilitazione: quale rapporto? Ital J Rehab Med MR. 2006;20:269–75.
24. Bø K. Pelvic floor muscle training in treatment of female stress urinary incontinence, pelvic organ prolapse and sexual dysfunction. World J Urol. 2012;30:437–43.
25. Aponte MM, Rosenblum N. Repair of pelvic organ prolapse: what is the goal? Curr Urol Rep. 2014;15:385.
26. Samuelsson EC, Victor FT, Tibblin G, et al. Signs of genital prolapse in a Swedish population of women 20 to 59 years of age and possible related factors. Am J ObstetGynecol. 1999;180:299–305.
27. Ashton-Miller JA, DeLancey JO. Functional anatomy of the female pelvic floor. In: Bo K, Berghmans B, Morkved S, Kampen MV, editors. Evidence-based physical therapy for the pelvic floor. St Louis: Elsevier; 2007. p. 19–33.
28. Slieker-ten Hove M, Pool-Goudzwaard A, Eijkemans M, et al. Pelvic floor muscle function in a general population of women with and without pelvic organ prolapse. Int Urogynecol J. 2010;21:311–9.
29. DeLancey JO. The hidden epidemic of pelvic floor dysfunction: achievable goals for improved prevention and treatment. Am J Obstet Gynecol. 2005;192:1488–95.
30. Chen L, Ashton-Miller JA, Hsu Y, et al. Interaction among apical support, levator ani impairment, and anterior vaginal wall prolapse. Obstet Gynecol. 2006;108:324–32.
31. Alas AN, Anger JT. Management of apical pelvic organ prolapse. Curr Urol Rep. 2015;16:33.
32. Culligan PJ. Nonsurgical management of pelvic organ prolapse. Obstet Gynecol. 2012;119:852–60.
33. Piya-Anant M, Therasakvichya S, Leelaphatanadit C, et al. Integrated health research program for the Thai elderly: prevalence of genital prolapse and effectiveness of pelvic floor exercise to prevent worsening of genital prolapse in elderly women. J Med Assoc Thai. 2004;85:509–15.
34. Ghroubi S, Kharrat O, Chaari M, et al. Effect of conservative treatment in the management of low-degree urogenital prolapse. Ann Readapt Med Phys. 2008;51:96–102.
35. Hagen S, Stark D, Glazener C, et al. A randomized controlled trial of pelvic floor muscle training for stages I and II pelvic organ prolapse. Int Urogynecol J Pelvic Floor Dysfunct. 2009;20(1):45–51.
36. Stüpp L, Resende AP, Oliveira E, et al. Pelvic floor muscle training for treatment of pelvic organ prolapse: an assessor-blinded randomized controlled trial. Int Urogynecol J. 2011;22:1233–9.
37. Alves FK, Riccetto C, Adami DB, et al. A pelvic floor muscle training program in postmenopausal women: a randomized controlled trial. Maturitas. 2015;81:300–5.
38. Brækken IH, Majida M, Ellström Engh M, et al. Can pelvic floor muscle training improve sexual function in women with pelvic organ prolapse? A randomized controlled trial. J Sex Med. 2015;12:470–80.
39. Wiegersma M, Panman CM, Kollen BJ, et al. Effect of pelvic floor muscle training compared with watchful waiting in older women with symptomatic mild pelvic organ prolapse: randomised controlled trial in primary care. BMJ. 2014;349:g7378.
40. Kashyap R, Jain V, Singh A. Comparative effect of 2 packages of pelvic floor muscle training on the clinical course of stage I-III pelvic organ prolapsed. Int J Gynecol Obstet. 2013;121:69–73.
41. Miedel A, Tegerstedt G, Maehle-Schmidt M, et al. Non obstetric risk factors for symptomatic pelvic organ prolapse. Obstet Gynecol. 2009;113:1089–97.
42. Saks EK, Harvie HS, Asfaw TS, et al. Clinical significance of obstructive defecatory symptoms in women with pelvic organ prolapse. Int J Gynaecol Obstet. 2010;111(3):237–40.
43. Braekken IH, Majida M, Ellstrom Engh M, et al. Pelvic floor function is independently associated with pelvic organ prolapse. BJOG. 2009;116:1706–14.
44. Whitcomb EL, Lukacz ES, Lawrence JM, et al. Prevalence and degree of bother from pelvic floor disorders in obese women. Int Urogynecol J Pelvic Floor Dysfunct. 2009;20(3):289–94.
45. Washington BB, Erekson EA, Kassis NC, et al. The association between obesity and stage II or greater prolapse. Am J Obstet Gynecol. 2010;202:503.
46. Braekken I, Majida M, Engh ME, et al. Morphological changes after pelvic floor muscle training measured by 3-dimensional ultrasonography. Obstet Gynecol. 2010;115:317–24.

47. Panman C, Wiegersma M, Kollen BJ, et al. Two-year effects and cost-effectiveness of pelvic floor muscle training in mild pelvic organ prolapse: a randomised controlled trial in primary are. BJOG. 2016. https://doi.org/10.1111/1471-0528.13992.
48. Hagen S, Stark D, Glazener C, et al. Individualised pelvic floor muscle training in women with pelvic organ prolapse (POPPY): a multicentre randomised controlled trial. Lancet. 2014;383:796–806.
49. Li C, Gong Y, Wang B. The efficacy of pelvic floor muscle training for pelvic organ prolapse: a systematic review and meta-analysis. Int Urogynecol J. 2016;27(7):981–92.
50. Bø K, Hilde G, Stær-Jensen J, et al. Postpartum pelvic floor muscle training and pelvic organ prolapse—a randomized trial of primiparous women. Am J Obstet Gynecol. 2015;212(1):38. e1–7.
51. Glazener CMA, McArthur C, Hagen S, et al. Twelve-year follow-up of conservative management of postnatal urinary and fecal incontinence and prolapsed outcomes: randomised controlled trial. BJOG. 2014;121:112–20.
52. Hullfish KL, Bovbjerg VE, Gurka MJ, et al. Surgical versus nonsurgical treatment of women with pelvic floor dysfunction: patient centered goals at 1 year. J Urol. 2008;179(6):2280–5.
53. Barber MD, Brubaker L, Burgio KL, et al. Comparison of 2 transvaginal surgical approaches and perioperative behavioral therapy for apical vaginal prolapse: the OPTIMAL randomized trial. JAMA. 2014;311:1023–34.
54. Pauls R, Crisp CC, Novicki K, et al. Pelvic floor physical therapy: impact on quality of life 6 months after vaginal reconstructive surgery. Female Pelvic Med Reconstr Surg. 2013;1:34–9.
55. McClurg D, Hilton P, Dolan L, et al. Pelvic floor muscle training as an adjunct to prolapse surgery: a randomised feasibility study. Int Urogynecol J. 2014;25:883–91.
56. Hagen S, Stark D. Conservative prevention and management of pelvic organ prolapse in women. Cochrane Database Syst Rev. 2011;12:CD003882.

Pessary: A Rediscovered Tool

Elena Cattoni, Paola Sorice, and Linda Leidi-Bulla

7.1 Evolution of Pessary Usage

Pelvic organ prolapse (POP) is a common pelvic floor disorder in women. Its diagnosis is associated with significant symptomatic distress and impaired quality of life (QoL). POP symptoms include vaginal bulging and pelvic heaviness. Up to 69% of women with a genital descensus also have another concurrent pelvic floor disorder, such as any kind of urinary, fecal, and/or sexual dysfunctions [1, 2], which often depend upon the type and stage of prolapse.

The aim of any POP treatment is to relieve the discomfort reported by our patients; therefore regardless the result of doctor's physical examination, the absence of specific symptoms does not require any treatment, unless clinical follow up. However, in addition to the possibility of a surgical management, the patient's symptomatology may find improvement, thanks to the use of conservative therapies, like vaginal pessaries, pelvic floor muscle training, and lifestyle advices.

Until the early nineteenth century, before the advent of asepsis and the improvement of surgical and anesthetic techniques, pessary was considered the main therapeutic device for symptomatic pelvic organ descensus. In contrast with the innovations of the different pelvic reconstructive surgery techniques, over the years, there have not been major changes in the practice of pessary use, but despite this, it still remains the most common nonsurgical treatment.

The word "pessary" comes from a Greek word *pessós*, meaning an oval stone used in checkers-like game initially inserted into the uterus of camels to prevent

E. Cattoni (✉) · L. Leidi-Bulla
Department of Gynecology and Obstetrics, Regional Hospital of Lugano, EOC,
Lugano, Switzerland
e-mail: elenacattoni@hotmail.it, cattoni@centromedico.ch

P. Sorice
Department of Gynecology and Obstetrics, Ospedale Giuseppe Fornaroli, Magenta, Italy

© Springer International Publishing AG, part of Springer Nature 2018
V. Li Marzi, M. Serati (eds.), *Management of Pelvic Organ Prolapse*,
Urodynamics, Neurourology and Pelvic Floor Dysfunctions,
https://doi.org/10.1007/978-3-319-59195-7_7

Fig. 7.1 Reduction of
vaginal prolapsed by using
natural objects [6]

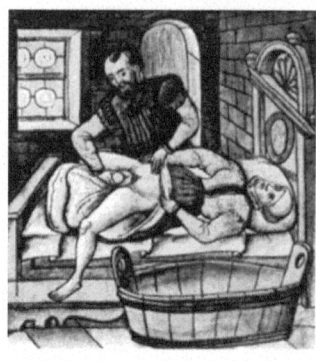

conception [3, 4]. Pessaries, intended as passive medical devices designed to support the vaginal walls and prevent any pelvic organ herniation, have been mentioned since the first recorded medical writings, as early as the fifth century BC, even by Hippocrates (Fig. 7.1). The earliest "pessaries" were described by two Greek physicians: Polybus advised to place a half pomegranate in the vagina, while Soranus a linen tampon soaked with astringent vinegar and a piece of beef [3]. Anyway, the first purpose-made devices have been actually designed only from the sixteenth century. Different materials have been used throughout the centuries: starting from natural objects, including fruits, wax-covered cork, or sponge until natural metals such as gold, silver, and brass. These devices sometimes have also been attached to perineal strap with a belt worn around the waist to support the vaginal walls [5].

7.2 Pessary for Pelvic Organ Prolapse

The **purpose** of the pessary prescription is to use an intravaginal device that conservatively avoids the protrusion of the pelvic viscera in the vagina to prevent worsening of the anatomical defect, reduce the frequency and severity of symptoms, and avoid or delay surgery.

There are very few **contraindications** to their use, which enables clinicians to potentially prescribe pessary to the majority of patients with a diagnosis of genital prolapse. Women should be excluded from the use of intravaginal devices in case of any undiagnosed abnormal vaginal bleeding or if they show a limited mobility that could hinder either their ability to self-management or their compliance with further follow-up visits. Indeed, the main contraindication for pessary fitting is the likelihood of noncompliance with follow-up, which is important to avoid further complications. Therefore any condition, such as dementia or the absence of an adequate support network, that could be responsible of neglected pessaries should be taken into account before prescribing them.

Moreover, severe vaginal atrophy, persistent vaginal erosions or ulcerations, and active vulvovaginal infections may be relative contraindications until they do not recover.

Indications for pessary use include contraindications for surgery either in surgical candidates at high risk due to their medical status or in young women who have not completed childbearing. Besides, many women could wish a nonsurgical management because of their fear for surgery [7, 8] or the lack of confidence in surgical results possibly due to previous history of unsuccessful surgical repair.

Pessary could also be recommended as a diagnostic tool to predict POP surgical outcome since the evidence [9] suggest that the insertion test is a reliable method to unmask occult stress urinary incontinence and to predict its occurrence after POP repair: it could be either fit during the urodynamic preoperative work-up [10] or as a temporary measure while awaiting for surgery [11].

The prevalence of prolapse during pregnancy is unknown. Pessary could temporarily relieve prolapse symptoms until delivery or until prolapse improvement, helped by a progressive increase in size of the gravid uterus. In case of its use for reducing pelvic prolapse during pregnancy, mixed efficacy results have been published [12].

Even if, the main reason for pessary use is to give patients an option for the relief of POP symptoms, some devices have been specifically designed for the treatment of stress urinary incontinence (SUI) whose diagnosis can be or not associated with the presence of POP. There is limited evidence from randomized controlled trials (RCTs) to judge whether their use for this specific indication is better than no treatment or whether one device is more effective than others in obtaining relief of incontinence symptoms [13]. A multidisciplinary survey conducted in the UK noted a considerable difference in the proportion of professionals providing pessary care for women with POP (100%) and those with SUI (55.7%) [14].

Another different use of pessary includes an attempt to avoid vaginal wind that can occur with a gaping vagina due to weak pelvic floor muscles [15].

Nowadays silicon-made pessary should be used in daily practice. Silicon offers many advantages due to its favorable characteristics: nonabsorbent properties in relation to secretions and odors; a long half-life and resistance to autoclave, allowing repeated cleaning; and also being inert, hypoallergenic, and non-cancerogenic [4, 5]. Since that rubber- and latex-made pessaries are used less and less, while selecting the proper pessary, its style and its dimensions are the main features to consider. Thanks to patient's individual variables and the presence of a wide variety of pessary shapes and sizes, it is possible to individualize their choice. The variables that can influence the picking process are sexual activity, type and degree of prolapse, and ability to self-management and to attend follow-ups.

Intravaginal devices for POP can be mainly divided into two different **types**: support or space filling pessaries. There is a multitude of models and forms (Fig. 7.2) of vaginal pessaries on the market, but only few models are actually widely used (Fig. 7.3) [16]. Possible explanations for this limited use could be the requirement of more training to gain greater confidence, the financial implications of introduction of newer devices, or simply a general reluctance by some clinicians [14].

Support pessaries uphold the prolapsed structure using a spring mechanism since they are thought to fit between the posterior fornix and behind the pubis. The ring is the most commonly support pessary used [14, 17] and it is usually advocated

Fig. 7.2 Various types of pessaries. (A) Ring. (B) Shaatz. (C) Gellhorn. (D) Gellhorn. (E) Ring with support. (F) Gellhorn. (G) Risser. (H) Smith. (I) Tandem cube. (J) Cube. (K) Hodge with knob. (L) Hodge. (M) Gehrung. (N) Incontinence dish with support. (O) Donut. (P) Incontinence ring. (Q) Incontinence dish. (R) Hodge with support. (S) Inflatoball (latex) (Courtesy of Milex Products, a division of Cooper Surgical, Trumbull, Connecticut)

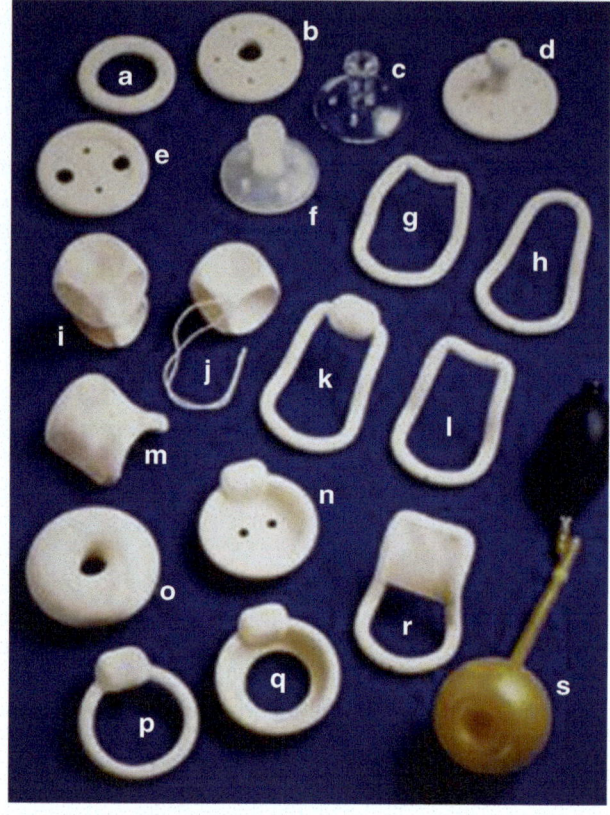

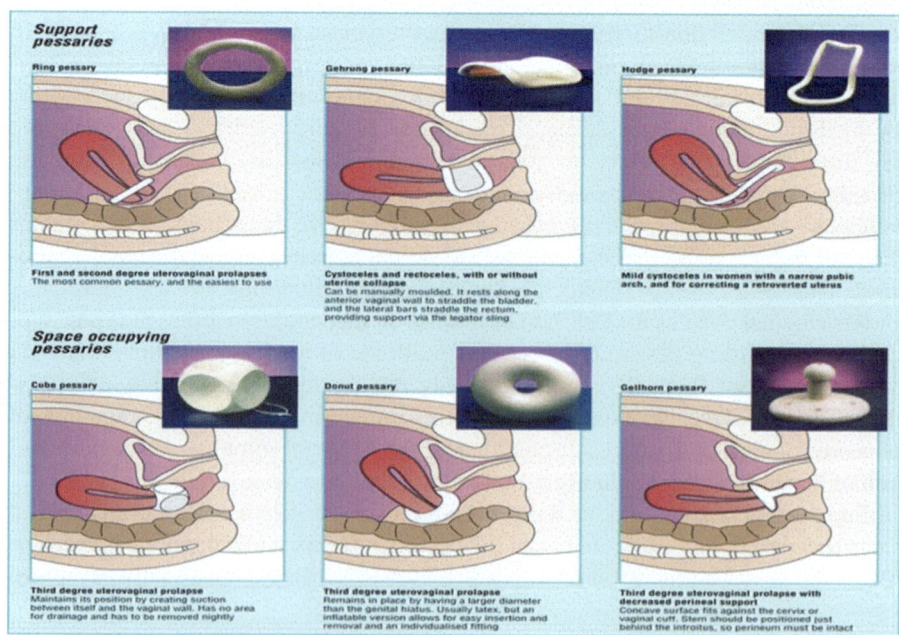

Fig. 7.3 Variety of pessaries mostly used [16]

for the initial fitting. It is considered to be the easiest to use for both the physician and the patient, especially when self-management is expected [18, 19]. Since it is open, it allows penetrative sexual intercourse but also the drainage of vaginal secretion; therefore it gives the patients the possibility to retain the ring in the vagina for longer periods, without the need of daily removal [3]. Conversely, it has the disadvantage that the cervix could protrude through the ring. Dish pessary has a central perforated support diaphragm which can be useful in case of procidentia, even if the closed structure prevents sexual intercourse if pessary is not removed from the vagina. The incontinence ring pessary is fitted in the same way, with an additional knob that should be situated suburethral behind the symphysis, ideally at the level of the urethro-vesical junction.

Space-filling devices use different mechanism to support the vaginal walls, since they stay in place without using the symphysis: Gellhorn and cube retain their position by suction of their surface on the vaginal walls, while donut merely occupies the vaginal space, as long as the pessary diameter is larger than the genital hiatus (GH). Space fillers have traditionally been used for the treatment of bigger prolapse stage [20, 21] or after the failure in the positioning of a support pessary. Due to the greater friction or to the suction mechanism against the vaginal wall, they are more at risk of causing vaginal erosion, and for this reason it is necessary a daily self-management or more frequent follow-up visits [22, 23]. Sexual intercourses are not allowed with the pessary in place, but many women feel at ease in removing it before intercourse [22, 24].

While there are identifiable trends in pessary use, there is no clear consensus regarding the indications for support pessaries compared with space-filling ones [22, 25] or the use of a single pessary for all support defects compared with tailoring the pessary to the specific defect [17] and patients' characteristics [26]. Usually clinicians rely on guidelines of factory manufacturers, expert opinions, personal experience, or patients' preference [5]. There is limited evidence from randomized controlled trials [25] to judge whether their use is better than other treatment, either conservative [27] or surgical, or to evaluate the superiority of one device on another for the relief of symptoms [25]. The PESSRI study is the only randomized crossover trial that has compared symptoms relief and change in life impact for women using the ring with support or Gellhorn pessaries: both were effective in determining statistically and clinically significant improvements in the majority of the Pelvic Floor Distress Inventory (PFDI) and many Pelvic Floor Impact Questionnaire (PFIQ) scales, but no clinically significant differences between the two pessaries were found [25].

Sizes of different devices won't be discussed in detail as they may slightly change with the pessary choice brand. The pessary fitting process cannot be made scientifically, since the identification of specific vaginal measures to adapt to a specific type of pessary is not possible [28], but it follows a trial-and-error process. For those women who have not retained the pessary or when the pessary is uncomfortable, a further trial with a different size or type of pessary is recommended. It has been described the chance to try an average of 3.5 pessaries, for each patient [29].

At initial visit the patients should be examined in both the litotomic and the standing position, at rest and straining. Pessary should be sufficiently large as not to fall out, but not so large to cause the patients any sensation of pressure, discomfort, or pain. Therefore, the best size for a given patient is the smallest one that will not fall out [30]. Usually the right size allows the examining finger to be passed freely all around the device. The right-fitted pessary should neither be expelled during Valsalva maneuver nor obstruct the bladder nor the bowel while emptying. After the first insertion, an adequate pathway of close monitoring and review must be scheduled.

7.3   Efficacy

Pessary use is associated with significant clinical improvement [19, 31, 32] not only in POP symptoms but also in bowel [33, 34] and urinary symptoms, such as voiding problems, frequency, urinary urgency, and urinary urgency incontinence [34–36]. However, 4–21% of women with no prior urinary symptoms developed problems with voiding dysfunction within 2 months of pessary placement [37], and occult stress urinary incontinence may be unmasked [22, 35, 38]. Satisfaction with the pessary usage and the absence of bothersome vaginal symptoms are associated with improvement in QoL [6] and with higher sexual function score in women [24]. Sexual function is not negatively affected by pessary use [24, 34]; therefore women should be adequately counseled and followed up in all their concerns.

Anyway, the data currently available in the literature regarding the efficacy of the pessary as a therapeutic tool have limited scientific value: most published papers are retrospective, and the follow-up period is mostly short, less than 12 months; results obtained from cohort studies, both retrospective and prospective, are not easily comparable due to little use of validated questionnaires to investigate pelvic floor dysfunction symptoms [19, 25, 32, 34] and due to different definitions of success and different management protocols and type of devices used; moreover comparison with other prolapsed therapies is rare and not yet assessed in a randomized controlled trial (RCT) [6, 27, 39].

Even if there are currently no clear evidence-based guidelines on the management of women with pessaries that have been endorsed by a recognized urogynecological association [40], pessary still remains a simple, inexpensive, viable, and practical option. Surgery of genital prolapse is frequent and often necessary: it is estimated that the lifetime risk of undergoing surgery for POP or urinary incontinence is 11% [41]. Thanks to the aging of population worldwide, there has been a renewed interest in the use of conservative treatment for POP, which is a valid alternative to surgery: Abdool and colleagues have demonstrated that, in a short-term follow-up, pessary could be equally effective compared to surgery in improving patients' symptoms [42]; however Mamik et al. have found that patients that underwent surgery have had significantly greater improvement in objective measures and a greater degree of success based on their self-defined goals [43].

Women could end up using their pessary only intermittently [44]. There are suggestions that pessaries may prevent progression of POP stage or result in improvement in its severity [4]: improved levator ani muscle function secondary to recovery from passive stretch induced by the pessary support of the pelvic organs [45–47] or local inflammation that lead to vaginal fibrosis may explain improvement in pessary users.

7.4 Patient Characteristics Associated with Pessary Choice

Different surveys conducted between gynecologists concluded that 87–98% of clinicians, both general practitioners and urogynecologists, use pessaries in their clinical practice [17, 26, 48] and 77% of them consider it as first-line therapy [26]. However a lack of consensus exists whether conservative therapies should always be attempted at first, considering the ease of use, the lack of major side effects when correctly handled and the low cost [21, 44].

A median of 2.4–5 pessaries is fitted every month with an average of 2.9 different types [14, 17]. Therefore, even if gynecologists widely use pessaries in their clinical practice, either they do not prescribe them often or women do not easily accept them. These data could explain why patients' enrollment in clinical studies could be challenging [49].

The choice of surgical compared with nonsurgical management should be made by the patients after a specific and adequate counseling that accurately addresses risks and benefits of both choices [30]. Even because when the option between surgery and conservative treatment is offered, the majority of women could choose to start from conservative management [8, 11, 17] either because they desired it since the beginning or because they changed their mind after counseling [7, 50]. In an insurance-based healthcare system, patients who are more likely to change their mind and choose for a conservative therapy are mostly those who cannot afford surgery, due to a lack of adequate insurance coverage [7, 50]. On the contrary, 75% of women who are scheduled for surgery could attempt a pessary trial because they prefer rapid symptoms relief over a long waiting list [7, 51]. However, women, whose first preference is for surgery at the time of pessary fitting, are more likely to discontinue pessary use [35].

Literature on pessaries is mainly focused on the treatment characteristics (patient satisfaction, successful fitting, discontinuation, efficacy, and complication rates), while factors influencing the choice of treatment itself, both by the patient and the physician, are much less studied [51], and results are often controversial and no consistent characteristics have been identified [38]. Even so, specific individual features could predict successful fitting and can be used for patient's counseling when faced in treatment choice. The reasons why patients discontinue pessary use after a first initial successful fitting may be significantly different than the reasons why they are not appropriately fitted. Success or failure may depend on appropriate pessary selection, patient characteristics, type of follow-up, training, and experience.

Twelve percent of gynecologists declares to reserve pessary as first-line therapy only for patients who refuse or are not candidates for pelvic surgery [26]. Women who prefer surgery usually are sexually active [8], have significantly more advanced

POP, and describe more severe pelvic dysfunction symptoms and impaired QoL at baseline [8, 17, 50–52]. However, we must take into account that it might not be a merely patient's decision, since the severity of the clinical picture might somehow influence the physician's counseling, which can consequently direct the patient to the surgical choice [7, 20, 51].

The age of the patient greatly influences the therapeutic choice. Literature suggests that pessaries are mostly prescribed to older women ($\geq$65 years old) [39], who are also more prone to accept this type of therapy and to continue to use it over time [8, 35, 44]. Younger patients are more likely to ultimately undergo surgery, whatever their initial desire may have been [8, 50]. In fact, even if it was previously described that the rate of prolapse surgery in younger patients was decreasing, more recent evidence demonstrates that they are more likely to opt for pelvic surgery [35]. This trend is probably helped by the increasing number of conservative reconstructive surgery attempts [53–55].

Moreover, many women decline vaginal pessary when they refer urinary incontinence to be more bothersome compare to prolapsed symptoms: in fact, the presence of concomitant stress urinary incontinence increases by 3.3 times the probability that the patient with prolapse demands surgery [51].

It is understandable that patients who failed to retain pessary would be more likely to choose for surgical treatment. There is not agreement in literature in what it is considered **successful pessary fitting**. There have been reported different percentages of success that reach up to 96.6% [11, 19, 29, 56–58]. In a 5-year prospective study, Lore and colleagues demonstrated that if pessary successfully treated POP symptoms at 4 weeks, 86.1% of women will continue the treatment over 5 years [11].

Many clinical variables have been addressed to understand what characteristics could potentially influence the fitting success rate: neither age [44], higher-stage POP [29, 44, 58], nor more bothersome POP symptoms have been associated with unsuccessful fitting [29, 58], implying that women with severe POP, either objectively or subjectively, should be not counseled against this type of conservative therapy. Instead, whether a history of previous hysterectomy or pelvic reconstructive surgery could fail initial pessary fitting is controversial [11, 19, 29, 58]. However, 42% of members of the American Urogynecologic Society (AUGS) consider previous pelvic surgery a contraindication for pessary use [26]: data addresses a higher unsuccessful fitting rate when surgery determines a shortening of the total vaginal length (TVL) 7 cm or less, a narrowing of the upper part of the vagina, and a GH/TVL ratio greater than 0.8–0.9 [19, 29, 35, 44, 58]. Anyhow, 36% of patients with a hysterectomy still have a successful fitting, and thus, these patients should still be offered this conservative therapy [58]. The presence of a posterior vaginal wall prolapse could also predict an unsuccessful pessary trial, but published data are mixed: while some authors attributed a greater unsuccessful rate to the weakening of rectovaginal fascia [44, 57], other researchers didn't find any statistical association between site of prolapse and risk of pessary failure [29, 58, 59]. Even a history of smoking has been associated with a greater difficulty in retaining the pessary in place, probably due to thinner vaginal mucosa that makes pessary more uncomfortable or to chronic coughing that could help pessary to fall out [29].

Pessary use was found to improve sexual function in some women [19, 34]: sexual activity is not correlated with an unsuccessful fitting [29], and pessary was found to be an acceptable long-term option in sexually active women [52]. Therefore, if women are sexually active should not be a deterrent to physicians when offering the use of pessary. Anyhow, patients who are more sexually active, those who avoid sexual activity because of prolapse, and those who feel that prolapse interferes with sexual satisfaction are more likely to opt for surgery [8].

Different studies report that **discontinuation rate** is 8–56% [8, 38, 50, 51]. The median time to pessary discontinuation is 5.1–5.8 years [38, 44]. After a period of conservative treatment, among who decide to remove the pessary, 71% of women undergo surgical repair, while 29% choose to suspend any further treatment [38].

Whether a patient continues or not to use pessary after initial fitting depends on how satisfied she is with the treatment [5, 22]. Specific objective and subjective treatment goals should be discussed with the patients in order to individualize the treatment options offered. Women affected by POP can have impaired self-body image. It is important to have the patients distinguish between "physical bother" and "mental bother": understanding patient's expectations allows physician to carefully manage them [30]. An optimal counseling should provide a realistic expectation for clinical outcome that a woman might expect from pessary use.

Dissatisfaction with the use of the pessary could be associated with inadequate symptoms relief [11, 44], discomfort [22, 29], or inability of carrying pessary [38, 48]. Patients who more frequently end up choosing a surgical repair within 1 year from the first fit are younger [29, 38, 50], and the principal reason advocated for stopping using the pessary is the appearance of de novo occult stress urinary incontinence [22, 35, 38], vaginal complications associated with recurrent discharge or erosion [11, 38], and dislike in the changing procedure [48].

7.5   Management

After attaining a good fit, the second step is educating the patient on how to wear and care for the device. An adjustment period eventually allows women to gain relief of symptoms and emotional distress in order to resume their daily lives [5, 7].

Speaking of pessary dealing, variables to consider include timing of follow-up after the initial fitting, the frequency of follow-up thereafter, use of replacement hormone therapy in postmenopausal women, the type of pessary to be placed, and any additional conservative options for unsuccessful pessary trials. Different survey of urogynecologists from around the world identifies wide patterns of advice and follow-up [14, 17, 26, 48]. Anyhow, pessary needs to be removed regularly and the vaginal mucosa checked for erosions.

After the first insertion, an adequate pathway of close monitoring and review must be scheduled: a follow-up visit after 1–2 weeks is advisable to check the pessary size and patient's symptoms [40]. Thereafter, most pessaries have been traditionally changed every 3–6 months, believing that regular changing prevents infections and erosions. However, there is no evidence that regular changing reduces rates of complications: Gorti et al. demonstrated a lack of differences in proportions of complications observed in 3-month (40.3%) and 6-month (35.2%) changing intervals, and it even tended to be decreased up to 12-month (18.5%) follow-up period [48]. Therefore they suggest that 6-month and probably up to 12-month intervals represent a safe and cost-effective regimen to follow up patients with vaginal pessaries [48].

Moreover, the evidence for or against pessary reuse after washing is minimal [23]. Descriptive data suggest that the contemporary prescription of local estrogens may be beneficial in successful pessary fitting or in maintenance of treatment with pessary [17, 26, 48, 60], but more evidence is needed about ongoing pessary management [39].

A multidisciplinary survey of pessary use practice showed that pessary care is predominantly undertaken by medical staff (96.8%), while few nurses (1.8%) and physiotherapists (1.4%) involved in the women's health field reported to have a role in pessary care [14]. Urogynecological providers who offer pessary fitting should counsel and work with their patients to develop an individualized and continuous treatment plan that includes appropriate care and follow-up.

Self-care is a central stronghold of contemporary healthcare policy. Only 53% of AUGS members teach all patients self-care, and 45% only teach those using support pessary [26]. A well-structured implementation program can promote training in self-insertion and care of different type of pessaries, even in rural and less wealthy communities where access to surgical care is inadequate [7, 61].

Since there is no research to support an optimum routine, neither for self-management nor for outpatient change, pessary care should be individualized on assessment of individual needs [40]. Healthcare teamwork, involving doctors and trained nurses [60], is desirable to provide the patient with a constant support that is useful not only for the decision process of the therapeutic choice but also in the management of the pessary, especially if self-management is eligible. Nurses can teach patients how to insert, remove, and maintain pessaries. An educated patient is much more satisfied with pessary treatment and better able to inform her provider if problems arise [5, 7]. This approach can help to prevent potential complications, including infection and erosion, and development of fistula. In case of impossible or refused self-management, due to women's physical limitations or embracement [23], a more frequent follow-up should be provided.

7.6 Complications

Pessary is usually considered to be a safe management option of POP. However, there are some complications, more frequent in long-term users, that can affect the patient's satisfaction. Most of them are not dangerous and easy to deal with since they can be treated with periodical removal and topical therapies. They are also less likely to occur in women who perform self-care [35, 60].

Increased vaginal discharge with odor is usually associated with higher rates of infections, and it is relatively common for pessary users: bacterial vaginosis (BV) was noted in 32% of pessary users, versus 10% of controls. The relative risk of developing BV in pessary users was 3.3 ((OR, 4.37; 95% CI, 2.15–9.32), $P = 0.0002$) [62].

The most common complication is vaginal erosion or ulceration: vaginal mucosa should always be checked for erosion at the time of follow-up visit since it has been reported in women after only 2 months of pessary use [63]. Ulceration rate varies between 2 and 24% [35, 56, 60]. The ring pessary is less likely than the Gellhorn or cube to cause erosion [22, 23, 35, 56, 60]. It is important to take into account that it has been described that in case of tissue erosion or ulceration, a fistula could occur even after the pessary removal [64]. Therefore in case of relatively simple complication, a strict follow-up is still required.

More severe but less common complications, usually related to neglected devices [63], are mainly described in case reports and include vesicovaginal fistula [64], ureterovaginal fistula [65, 66], rectovaginal fistula, and urological complications such as bladder outlet obstruction due to urethral compression or ureteral obstruction from pressure under the bladder trigone and consequently acute pyelonephritis [67], cervical incarceration, or impacted pessaries. Keeping a list of pessary users with their follow-up schedules in the office may be useful, so if a patient is hospitalized or has a change in mental status, the hospital or caregiver may be informed of the patient's pessary use [5].

Other considerations include the possible effect of pessary on pap smears. Neglected pessaries could produce metaplasia and dysplastic change in the squamous mucosa [68]. Vaginal cancer related to pessary use has been described [69–71]. All related cases of vaginal cancer in the literature occurred at the site of contact with the pessary and the vaginal wall [69, 70]. Researchers have not been able to relate cancers to chemical cancerogenesis; therefore they concluded that it could be mostly associated with chronic inflammations [69].

In conclusion, pessaries are a valid option for symptomatic POP; however, their use entered in everyday clinical practice without a comprehensive and evidence-based assessment of its effectiveness in relation to other therapies, both surgical and conservative. A recent Cochrane review [39] concluded there is no good-quality evidence available in literature to be able to structure practical guidelines on the correct use (indications, shape choice, type of follow-up, role of local estrogen therapy) of pessaries. To help physicians to guide the patients to an individualized therapeutic management of POP, there is the need for well-designed RCTs specifically addressing to compare the use of pessary with other modes of treatment such as expectant management (control group), surgery, or physical interventions [27] and also to compare different types of devices [25].

References

1. Lawrence JM, Luckacz ES, Nager CW, et al. Prevalence and co-occurrence of pelvic floor disorder in community-dwelling women. Obstet Gynecol. 2008;11(3):678–85.
2. Haylen BT, de Ridder D, Freeman RM, et al. An International Urogynecological Association (IUGA)/International Continence Society (ICS) joint report on the terminology for female pelvic floor dysfunction. Int Urogynecol J. 2010;29:4–20.

3. Oliver R, Thakar R, Sultan AH. The history and usage of the vaginal pessary: a review. Eur J Obstet Gynecol Reprod Biol. 2011;156(2):125–30.
4. Shah SM, Sultan AH, Thakar R. The history and evolution of pessaries for pelvic organ prolapse. Int Urogynecol J Pelvic Floor Dysfunct. 2006;17(2):170–5.
5. Atrip SD. Pessary use and management for pelvic organ prolapse. Obstet Gynecol Clin N Am. 2009;36:541–63.
6. Lamers BHC, Broekman BMW, Milani AL. Pessary treatment for pelvic organ prolapse and health-related quality of life: a review. Int Urogynecol J. 2011;22:637–44.
7. Sevilla C, Wieslander CK, Alas A, et al. The pessary process: Spanish-speaking Latinas' experience. Int Urogynecol J. 2013;24(6):939–46.
8. Kapoor DS, Thakar R, Sultan AH, et al. Conservative versus surgical management of prolapse: what dictates patient choice? Int Urogynecol J Pelvic Floor Dysfunct. 2009;20(10):1157–61.
9. Serati M, Giarenis I, Meschia M, et al. Role of urodynamics before prolapse surgery. Int Urogynecol J. 2015;26(2):165–8.
10. Visco AG, Brubaker L, Nygaard I, et al. The role of preoperative urodynamic testing in stress-continent women undergoing sacrocolpopexy: the Colpopexy and Urinary Reduction Effort (CARE) randomized surgical trial. Int Urogynecol J Pelvic Floor Dysfunct. 2008;19:607–14.
11. Lone F, Thakar R, Sultan AH, et al. A 5-year prospective study of vaginal pessary use for pelvic organ prolapse. Int J Gynaecol Obstet. 2011;114:56–9.
12. Rusavy Z, Bombieri L, Freeman RM. Procidentia in pregnancy: a systematic review and recommendations for practice. Int Urogynecol J. 2015;26(8):1103–9.
13. Lipp A, Shaw C, Glavind K. Mechanical devices for urinary incontinence in women. Cochrane Database Syst Rev. 2014;(12):CD001756. https://doi.org/10.1002/14651858.CD001756.pub6.
14. Bugge C, Hegen S, Thakar R. Vaginal pessaries for pelvic organ prolapse and urinary incontinence: a multidisciplinary survey of practice. Int Urogynecol J. 2013;24:1017–24.
15. Jeffrey S, Franco A, Fynes M. Vaginal wind: the cube pessary as a solution. Int Urogynecol J. 2008;19:1457.
16. Thakar R, Stanton S. Management of genital prolapse. BMJ. 2002;324:1258–62.
17. Pott-Grinstein E, Newcomber JR. Gynecologists' pattern of prescribing pessaries. J Reprod Med. 2001;46:205–8.
18. ACOG Committee on Practice Bulletins—Gynecology. ACOG Practice Bulletin No. 85: Pelvic organ prolapse.
19. Fernando RJ, Thakar R, Sultan AH, et al. Effect of vaginal pessaries on symptoms associated with pelvic organ prolapse. Obstet Gynecol. 2006;108(1):93–9.
20. Bash KL. Review of vaginal prolapse pessaries. Obstet Gynecol Surv. 2000;55(7):455–60.
21. Weber AM, Richter HE. Pelvic organ prolapse. Obstet Gynecol. 2005;106:615–34.
22. Nemeth Z, Nagy S, Ott J. The cube pessary: an underestimated treatment option for pelvic organ prolapse? Subjective 1-year outcomes. Int Urogynecol J. 2013;24:1695–701.
23. Khaja A, Freeman RM. How often should shelf/Gellhorn pessaries changed? A survey of IUGA urogynecologists. Int Urogynecol J. 2014;25:941–6.
24. Meriwether KV, Komesu YM, Craig E, et al. Sexual function and pessary management among women using a pessary for pelvic floor disorders. J Sex Med. 2015;12:2339–49.
25. Cundiff GW, Amundsen CL, Bent AE, et al. The PESSRI study: symptom relief outcomes of a randomized crossover trial of the ring and Gellhorn pessaries. Am J Obstet Gynecol. 2007;196(4):405.e1–8.
26. Cundiff WG, Weidner AC, Visco AG, et al. A survey of pessary use by members of the American Urogynecologic Society. Obstet Gynecol. 2000;95(6 pt 1):931–5.
27. Wiegersma M, Panman CMCR, Kollen BJ, et al. Pelvic floor muscle training versus watchful waiting or pessary treatment for pelvic organ prolapse (POPPS): design and participant baseline characteristics of two parallel pragmatic randomized controlled trials in primary care. Maturitas. 2014;77:168–73.
28. Nager CW, Richter HE, Nygaard I, et al. Incontinence pessaries: size, POPQ measures, and successful fitting. Int Urogynecol J Pelvic Floor Dysfunct. 2009;20(9):1023–8.

29. Geoffrion R, Zhang T, Lee T, et al. Clinical characteristics associated with unsuccessful pessary fitting outcomes. Female Pelvic Med Reconstr Surg. 2013;19(6):339–45.
30. Culligan PJ. Nonsurgical management of pelvic organ prolapse. Obstet Gynecol. 2012;119(4):852–60.
31. Barber MD, Walters MD, Cundiff GW. Responsiveness of the Pelvic Floor Distress Inventory (PFDI) and Pelvic Floor Impact Questionnaire (PFIQ) in women under-going vaginal surgery and pessary treatment for pelvic organ prolapse. Am J Obstet Gynecol. 2006;194(5):1492–8.
32. Komesu YM, Rogers RG, Rode MA, et al. Pelvic floor symptom changes in pessary users. Am J Obstet Gynecol. 2007;197:620.e1–6.
33. Brazell HD, Patel M, O'sullivan DM, et al. The impact of pessary use on bowel symptoms: one-year outcome. Female Pelvic Med Reconstr Surg. 2014;20(2):95–8.
34. Kuhn A, Bapst D, Stadlmayr W, et al. Sexual and organ function in patients with symptomatic prolapse: are pessaries helpful? Fertil Steril. 2009;91(5):1914–8.
35. Clemons JL, Aguilar VC, Tillinghast TA, et al. Patient satisfaction and changes in prolapse and urinary symptoms in women who were successfully fitted with a pessary for pelvic organ prolapse. Am J Obstet Gynecol. 2004;190:1025–9.
36. Donnelly MJ, Powell-Morgan S, Olsen AL, et al. Vaginal pessaries for the management of stress and mixed urinary incontinence. Int Urogynecol J. 2004;15:302–7.
37. Manchana T, Bunyavejchevin S. Impact on quality of life after ring pessary use for pelvic organ prolapse. Int Urogynecol J. 2012;2:873–7.
38. Friedman S, Sandhu C, Wang C, et al. Factors influencing long-term pessary use. Int Urogynecol J. 2010;21:673–8.
39. Bugge C, Adams EJ, Gopinath D, et al. Pessaries (mechanical devices) for pelvic organ prolapse in women. Cochrane Database Syst Rev. 2013;(2):CD004010. https://doi.org/10.1002/14651858.CD004010.pub3.
40. Continence Foundation of Australia and International Centre for Allied Health Evidence, University of South Australia. Guidelines for the use of support pessaries in the management of pelvic organ pro-lapse. 2012. http://w3.unisa.edu.au/cahe/Resources/GuidelinesiCAHE/Pessary%20Guidelines.pdf.
41. Luber KM, Boero S, Choe JY. The demographics of pelvic floor disorders: current observations and future projections. Am J Obstet Gynecol. 2001;184(7):1496–501.
42. Abdool Z, Thakar R, Sultan AH. Prospective evaluation of outcome of vaginal pessaries versus surgery in women with symptomatic pelvic organ prolapse. Int Urogynecol J. 2011;22:273–8.
43. Mamik MM, Rogers RG, Qualls CR, et al. Goal attainment after treatment in patients with symptomatic pelvic organ prolapse. Am J Obstet Gynecol. 2013;209(488):e1–5.
44. Ramsay S, Tu LM, Tannenbaum C. Natural history of pessary use in women aged 65-74 versus 75 years and older with pelvic organ prolapse: a 12-year study. Int Urogynecol J. 2016;27(8):1201–7. https://doi.org/10.1007/s00192-016-2970-3.
45. Handa VL, Jones M. Do pessaries prevent the progression of pelvic organ prolapse? Int Urogynecol J Pelvic Floor Dysfunct. 2002;13(6):349–51.
46. Bo K, Majida M, Ellstrom ME. Does a ring pessary in situ influence the pelvic floor muscle function of women with pelvic organ prolapse when tested in supine? Int Urogynecol J. 2012;23:573–7.
47. Jones K, Yang L, Lowder JL, et al. Effect of pessary use on genital hiatus measurements in women with pelvic organ prolapse. Obstet Gynecol. 2008;112(3):630–6.
48. Gorti M, Hundelist G, Simons A. Evaluation of vaginal pessary management: a UK-based survey. J Obstet Gynaecol. 2009;29(2):129–31.
49. Hagen S, Sinclair L, Glazener C, et al. A feasibility study for randomized controlled trial with pelvic organ prolapse. ICS Conference, Glasgow, UK. 2001. http://iwcsoffice.org/Abstracts/Publish/106/000616.pdf.
50. Sullivan SA, Davidson EWR, Bretscneider EM, et al. Patient characteristics associated with treatment choice for pelvic organ prolapse and urinary incontinence. Int Urogynecol J. 2016;27:811–6.

51. Chan SS, Cheung RY, Yiu KW, et al. Symptoms, quality of life and factors affecting women's treatment decisions regarding pelvic organ prolapse. Int Urogynecol J. 2012;23:1027–33.
52. Brincat C, Kenton K, Pat Fitzgerald M, et al. Sexual activity predicts continued pessary use. Am J Obstet Gynecol. 2004;191(1):198–200.
53. Korbly NB, Kassis NC, Good MM, et al. Patient preferences for uterine preservation and hysterectomy in women with pelvic organ prolapsed. Am J Obstet Gynecol. 2013;209(5):470e1–6.
54. Detollenaere RJ, denBoon J, Stekelenburg J, et al. Sacrospinous hysteropexy versus vaginal hysterectomy with suspension of the uterosacral ligaments in women with uterine prolapse stage 2 or higher: multicentre randomised non-inferiority trial. BMJ. 2015;351:h3717. https://doi.org/10.1136/bmj.h3717.
55. Rahmanou P, Price N Jackson SR. Laparoscopic hysteropexy versus vaginal hysterectomy for the treatment of uterovaginal prolapse: a prospective randomized pilot study. Int Urogynecol J. 2015;26(11):1687–94.
56. Clemons JL, Aguillar VC, Tillinghast TA, et al. Risk factors associated with an unsuccessful pessary fitting trial in women with pelvic organ prolapse. Am J Obstet Gynecol. 2004;190(2):345–50.
57. Yamada T, Matsubara S. Rectocele, but not cystocele, may predict unsuccessful pessary fitting. J Obstet Gynaecol. 2011;31(5):441–2.
58. Markle D, Skoczylas L, Goldsmith C, et al. Patients characteristics associated with successful pessary fitting. Female Pelvic Med Reconstr Surg. 2011;17(5):249–52.
59. Mutone MF, Terry C, Hale DS, et al. Factors which influence the short term success of pessary management of pelvic organ prolapse. Obstet Gynecol. 2005;193:89–94.
60. Hanson LM, Schultz J, Flood CG, et al. Vaginal pessaries in managing women with pelvic organ prolapsed and urinary incontinence: patient characteristics and factors contributing to success. Int Urogynecol J. 2006;17:155–9.
61. Fitchett JR, Bhatta S, Sherpa TY, et al. Non-surgical interventions for pelvic organ prolapsed in rural Nepal: a prospective monitoring and evaluation study. JSRM Open. 2015;6(12):2054270415608117. https://doi.org/10.1177/2054270415608117. eCollection 2015.
62. Alnaif B, Drutz HB. Bacterial vaginosis increases in pessary users. Int Urogynecol J. 2000;11:219–23.
63. Arias BE, Ridgeway B, Barber MD. Complications of neglected vaginal pessaries: case presentation and literature review. Int Urogynecol J Pelvic Floor Dysfunct. 2008;19(8):1173–8.
64. Penrose KJ, Tsokos N. Delayed vesicovaginal fistula after ring pessary usage. Int Urogynecol J. 2014;25:291–3.
65. Walker KF, Dasgupta J, Cust MP. A neglected shelf pessary resulting in a urethrovaginal fistula. Int Urogynecol J. 2011;22:1133–4.
66. Ambereen DF. Ureterovaginal fistula due to a cube pessary despite routine follow-up: but what is "routine"? J Obstet Gynaecol Res. 2014;40:2162–5.
67. Ho MP. Unilateral acute pyelonephritis associated with neglected pessary. J Am Geriatr Soc. 2011;59:1962–3.
68. Christ ML, Haja J. Cytological changes associated with vaginal pessary use with special reference to the presence of actinomyces. Acta Cytol. 1973;22(3):146–9.
69. Schraub S, Sun XS, Maingon PH, et al. Cervical and vaginal cancer associated with pessary use. Cancer. 1992;69:2505–9.
70. Martin C, Hong L, Siddighi S. What is hiding behind the pessary? Int Urogynecol J. 2013;24:873–5.
71. Jain A, Majoko F, Freites O. How innocent is the vaginal pessary? Two cases of vaginal cancer associated with the pessary use. J Obstet Gynaecol. 2006;26(8):829–30.

Fascial Surgical Repair for Prolapse

8

Michele Meschia

8.1 Introduction

This chapter focuses on fascial reconstructive surgical management of pelvic organ prolapse through vaginal approach. The primary aim of surgery is to restore the body's normal support structure while returning the prolapsed organ to its normal anatomic position and relieving or improving prolapse symptoms.

Depending on the extent and location of prolapse, surgery usually involves a combination of repairs addressing the vaginal apex, anterior and posterior vagina, and perineum. Therefore the classification of prolapse according to the separate compartments is arbitrary, since the vagina is a continuum, and prolapse of one compartment is often associated with prolapse of another.

There is a wide variety of surgical procedures available for prolapse repair. This indicates that there is a lack of consensus as to the optimal surgical approach.

Traditionally, operations to treat uterovaginal prolapse include hysterectomy to initiate the surgery even when no specific uterine disease is present; however, it remains unknown whether concomitant hysterectomy at the time of prolapse surgery is integral to the effective cure of this condition, and few randomized clinical trials of hysterectomy vs no hysterectomy have been done. Uterine preservation in women with uterovaginal prolapse is only considered if future fertility is desired, but there has been a recent questioning of this practice because gynecologists and patients in many countries do not routinely prefer or perform hysterectomies in prolapse repairs. More women are requesting uterine preservation for many other reasons, including issues of sexuality, body image, and personal and cultural preferences. It has been shown that 60% of women indicated they would decline a

M. Meschia
Department of Obstetrics and Gynecology, ASST Ovest Milanese, Ospedale "Fornaroli", Magenta, MI, Italy
e-mail: m.meschia@libero.it

© Springer International Publishing AG, part of Springer Nature 2018
V. Li Marzi, M. Serati (eds.), *Management of Pelvic Organ Prolapse*, Urodynamics, Neurourology and Pelvic Floor Dysfunctions, https://doi.org/10.1007/978-3-319-59195-7_8

hysterectomy if presented with an equally efficacious alternative to a hysterectomy-based prolapse repair [1].

Most procedures that aim to suspend the vaginal apex can be done with or without hysterectomy, although some important technical modifications are sometimes necessary. A review on this topic by Gutman and Maher [2] concluded that uterine preservation during surgery for uterovaginal prolapse may be an option in appropriately selected women who desire it. Although the risk of unanticipated pathology in asymptomatic women with prolapse is very low [3], uterine-sparing procedures are not appropriate for women with a history of cervical dysplasia, abnormal uterine bleeding, and postmenopausal bleeding or those who are at high risk for uterine malignancy.

8.2   Apical Compartment Repair

The apex is the keystone of pelvic organ support. Support of the apex must be assessed regardless of the presence or absence of the uterus. Without good suspension of the uterus or post-hysterectomy vaginal cuff, the anterior and posterior walls are exposed to intra-abdominal forces that drive these tissues toward the introitus. Because of the significant contribution of the apex to anterior vaginal support, the best surgical correction of the anterior and posterior walls may fail unless the apex is adequately supported [4, 5]. While recognition of apical defects is one of the biggest problems in the evaluation of pelvic support defects, surgical correction of the apex has several good options with relatively high success rates.

8.2.1   McCall Culdoplasty

In 1957, McCall described the technique of closing the deep cul-de-sac at the time of vaginal hysterectomy to prevent enterocele formation [6]. Since then, other surgeons have modified the procedure, incorporating the uterosacral ligaments for apical support. This is the most frequently performed technique to close the posterior vaginal cuff, especially in surgical interventions for moderate POP cases involving vaginal hysterectomy.

The modified McCall culdoplasty is performed by placing one or two delayed absorbable suture through one of the uterosacral ligaments, incorporating the cul-de-sac peritoneum and vaginal cuff, and placing the final suture through the opposite uterosacral ligament [7]. It is uncertain if nonabsorbable sutures provide higher rates of cure; they do however result in more suture erosions [8]. Many authorities advocate using this procedure as part of every vaginal hysterectomy, even in the absence of prolapse, to minimize future formation of apical prolapse (Fig. 8.1).

Despite the frequency of this procedure, literature regarding outcomes is scarce. A small retrospective study ($n = 62$ per group) compared McCall culdoplasty to sacrospinous ligament suspension and found no difference in recurrences (15%) up to 9 years after the procedure [9]. The Mayo Clinic demonstrated 82%

Fig. 8.1 Modified McCall culdoplasty: sutures goes through the vaginal apex including both the uterosacral ligaments and the peritoneum

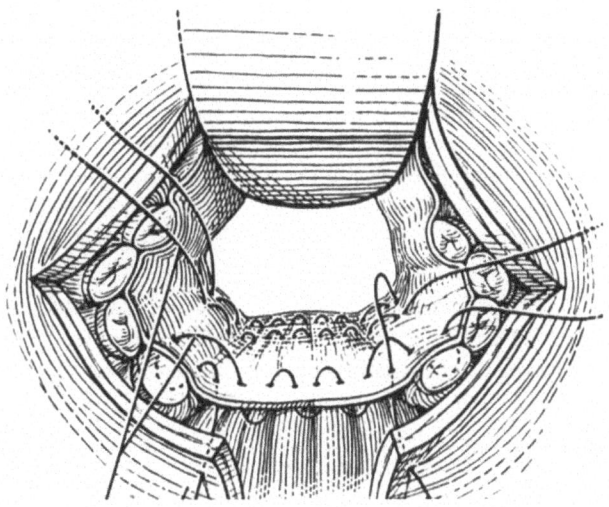

patient satisfaction and a reoperation rate of 5.2% in a larger retrospective study (n = 693) [10].

Risks of McCall's culdoplasty include ureteral obstruction or injury. Cystoscopy should be recommended intraoperatively with intravenous injection of indigo carmine or methylene blue to confirm ureteral patency.

Recently a large retrospective study has been published comparing the modified McCall culdoplasty with the high uterosacral ligament vaginal vault suspension (USLs) at the time of vaginal hysterectomy [11]. A total of 339 patients were evaluated at a mean follow-up of 26 months. Anatomical outcomes in terms of recurrence of prolapse at any site and reoperation rate did not show any statistically significant difference (20.9% and 1.4% vs. 15.3% and 1.6%, respectively). Rate of ureteral injuries was low both in McCall and USLs (1.9% and 0.8%, respectively).

8.2.2   Sacrospinous Ligament Fixation

The sacrospinous ligament fixation (SSLF) is one of the most frequently reported procedures for apical repair, in particular for vault prolapse. It is performed mainly unilaterally and no evidence exists on better outcomes if the procedure is done bilaterally. SSLF can be performed also at the end of vaginal hysterectomy in cases of severe uterine prolapse (stage ≥ III) or preserving the uterus by fixating the cervix to the ligament. Access to the sacrospinous ligament can be through a posterior vaginal dissection, through the apex, or by an anterior approach.

The posterior approach is the most popular and often requires the dissection and the high closure of an associated enterocele sac. The pararectal space is then entered by blunt dissection after mobilizing the rectum medially and the sacrospinous ligament identified after palpation of the ischial spine, as it courses from the ischial spine to the sacrum.

Optimal suture placement is 1.5–2.0 cm medial to the ischial spine to avoid damages to the pudendal neurovascular bundle, and no consensus exists regarding the number and type of sutures; commonly between one and three sutures are passed through the ligament with a combination of delayed absorbable and nonabsorbable materials.

The introduction into clinical practice of different transvaginal suture-capturing devices made the procedure safer, easier, and faster as the dissection of the pararectal space is limited and there is no longer need of positioning of vaginal retractors (Fig. 8.2).

It is important that the vagina comes into contact with the sacrospinous ligament and no suture bridge exists, to avoid any suture traction on the ligament (Fig. 8.3).

Current data is mainly observational, retrospective, and limited to anatomical results but suggests that this procedure is effective and safe. Several case series reported excellent success rates for correcting apical prolapse, although high rates of anterior vaginal prolapse have been reported too [12]. Posterior deflection of the vaginal axis with sacrospinous ligament fixation has been usually considered the reason for anterior recurrences, but lack of establishing continuity between anterior and apical compartments, especially in cases of vault prolapse, may be the stronger predictor.

Objectively, Barber and Maher [13] reported rates of 2.4–19% for anatomical recurrence, with the anterior wall as the most frequent site for recurrence. The OPTIMAL trial (Operations and Pelvic Muscle Training in the Management of Apical Support Loss) RCT study, comparing sacrospinous fixation and high uterosacral ligament vaginal vault suspension, found recurrent anterior wall prolapse beyond the hymen in 13.7% of cases [14]. Functionally, this anterior vaginal wall descent has been reported most often as an asymptomatic recurrence, which requires

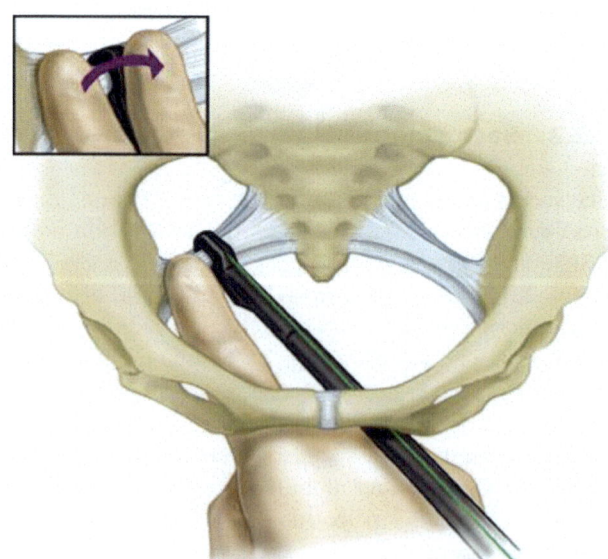

Fig. 8.2 Sacrospinous ligament anchoring with suture-capture devices

Fig. 8.3 Direct attachment
of the vaginal apex to the
sacrospinous ligament

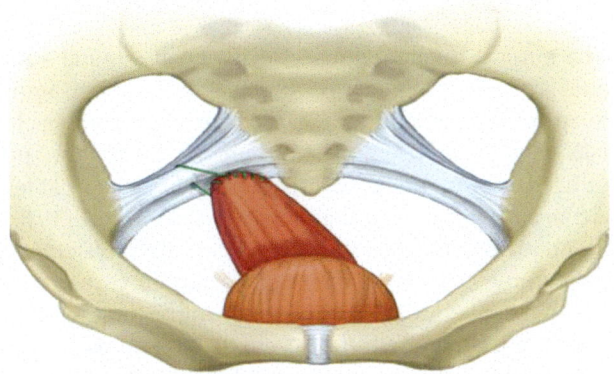

treatment only in 3–5% of patients undergoing SSLF [15]. Few studies focused on functional results. Symptomatic relief of 80–99% has been reported by different retrospective and prospective studies [12, 13, 15]. Postoperative buttock pain on the side on which the sacrospinous suspension has been performed can occur. This is probably related to compression of the levator ani nerve that runs through the coccygeus-sacrospinous ligament and can be more bothersome when sacrospinous hysteropexy is performed. However pain resolves usually within the course of the first month with the use of anti-inflammatory agents.

8.2.3   Iliococcygeus Fixation

Iliococcygeus fixation (ICF) provides attachment of the vaginal apex to the iliococcygeus muscle and fascia, usually bilaterally. The dissection to the area of the ischial spine is approached from a midline posterior vaginal incision. The rectovaginal fascia is freed from the vagina with sharp dissection and continued to the pelvic sidewall.

Using the ischial spine as the landmark for identifying the sacrospinous ligament medially and posteriorly and the iliococcygeus fascia anteriorly and caudal, a delayed absorbable suture is placed and attached to the vaginal apex.

A prospective nonrandomized matched case-control study, comparing ICF and SSLF, showed no significant difference in objective and subjective success rate or subsequent development of anterior vaginal wall prolapse [16].

Recently a prospective study on 44 patients, followed for a mean of 5 years after iliococcygeus fixation, showed subjective and objective success rates of 88.6% and 84.1%, respectively. The only preoperative independent risk factor for recurrence was stage IV vault descent [17].

Finally, a prospective nonrandomized trial, comparing the efficacy and safety of ICF and abdominal sacro-colpopexy in patients with vaginal vault prolapse, found a similar success rate in objective and functional results. Operative time was significantly shorter but median blood loss higher in the ICF group [18].

8.2.4 Uterosacral Ligament Vaginal Vault Suspension

The purpose of the uterosacral ligament vaginal vault suspension (USLs) is to attach a strong segment of the USL to the rectovaginal and pubocervical fascia. Suspending the vault at or above the level of the ischial spines usually provides adequate vaginal length and support. Until now, published descriptions have utilized two or more absorbable and nonabsorbable sutures in each ligament. According to the technique described by Shull [19], intraperitoneal exposure is accomplished through the vaginal cuff after hysterectomy or through a transverse colpotomy incision at the vaginal cuff in cases of vaginal vault prolapse. The bowel must be packed out of the operative field with long gauze to allow identification of USL on each side. A gentle traction with an Allis clamp is exerted on the caudal part of the ligament, and triple transfixion of USL is performed bilaterally with a monofilament number 0 delayed absorbable suture. The lowest suture is placed at the level of the ischial spine, and the two following are placed 1 cm above each. In total, six sutures are positioned. Then the suspending sutures are attached sequentially to the anterior and posterior leaves of the vaginal cuff, including the peritoneum. The most distal USL sutures are passed laterally, the proximal ones medially, and the intermediates ones between the previous ones. All sutures are tightened in order to close both the pouch of Douglas and the vaginal cuff (Fig. 8.4).

While performing USL suspensions, surgeons must have a high level of suspicion for ureteral injuries. Performing an intraoperative cystoscopy is an absolute necessity.

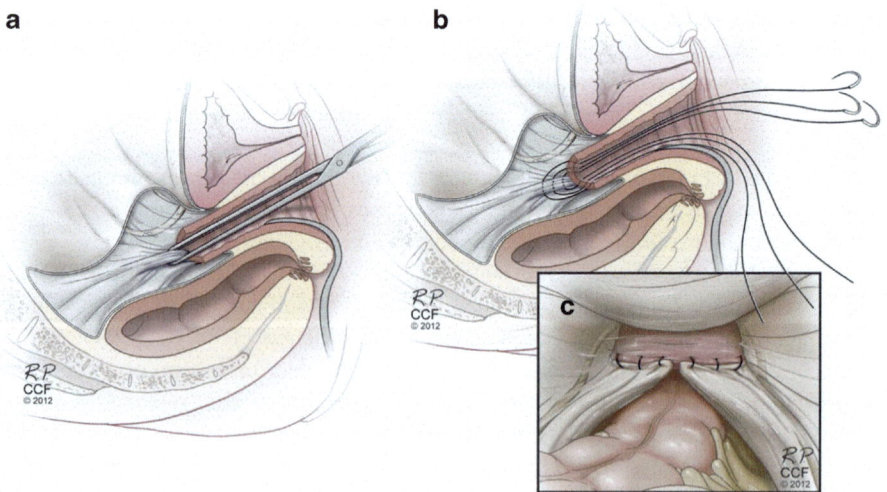

Fig. 8.4 Three pairs of sutures are placed along both uterosacral ligaments. (**a**) The uterosacral ligament at about the level of the ischial spine is grasped with an Allis clamp. (**b**) Three sutures are placed through the ipsilateral uterosacral ligament and then through the vaginal apex. (**c**) Sutures are placed bilaterally and tied, suspending the apex (Illustration by Ross Papalardo. Reprinted with permission, Cleveland Clinic Center for Medical Art & Photography 2010–2012. All rights reserved)

Published literature has shown good outcomes with USL suspension with reported success rates between 85 and 96% [14, 19–21]. Unfortunately, definitions of success differ, and direct comparisons of studies are difficult. Silva et al. [21] found that with 5-year follow-ups approximately 15.3% of patients had stage 2 or greater prolapse in one or more compartments. Only 2.8% of patients had recurrent apical prolapse.

The only randomized controlled trial for the USLs procedure (OPTIMAL trial) compared outcomes for USLs and SSLF with or without perioperative behavioral and pelvic floor muscle therapy in women who underwent surgery for apical vaginal prolapse. Anatomical and functional outcomes were not significantly different between procedures [14].

Recently a retrospective study on 20 patients who underwent transvaginal USLs, while preserving the uterus, reported anatomical recurrence in 5 subjects (25%) with a reoperation rate of 15% at a mean follow-up of 33 months [22].

8.3   Anterior Compartment Repair

Anterior vaginal prolapse has traditionally been repaired with anterior colporrhaphy, where the vaginal epithelium is separated from the underlying fibromuscular connective tissue (pubocervical fascia). Dissection must be forwarded laterally reaching the margin of the descending ischio-pubic bone, followed by midline plication of the pubocervical fascia. Typically delayed absorbable suture is used to reduce the risk of vaginal erosion, but some experts choose to use permanent suture material depending on the quality of the patient's tissues. This plication can be done in two layers if the defect is large. The excess mucosa is then trimmed, and the mucosa is closed using delayed absorbable sutures in a running fashion [23] (Figs. 8.5 and 8.6).

Attention must be given to reestablish continuity between anterior and apical compartment by suturing the proximal edge of the pubocervical fascia to the uterosacral-cardinal ligament complex or in cases of uterus preservation to the cervical ring.

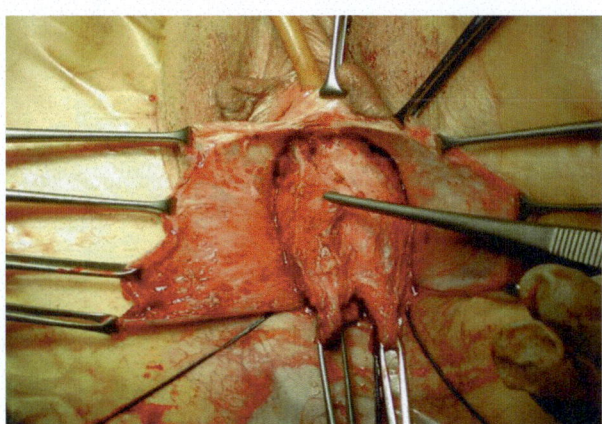

Fig. 8.5 Dissection of the pubocervical fascia from the vaginal epithelium extended laterally

Fig. 8.6 Midline fascia
plication with interrupted
stiches

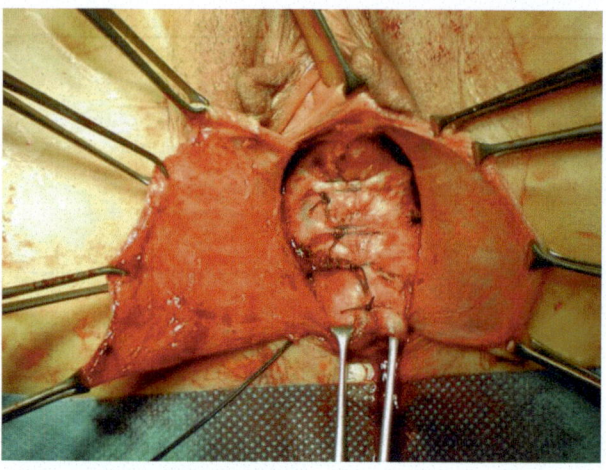

When a clearly demonstrable lateral defect exists, a vaginal paravaginal repair can be accomplished by entering the paravesical space and suturing the lateral edge of the pubocervical fascia to the arcus tendineus fasciae pelvis (white line) with a series of three to five absorbable or nonabsorbable sutures [24]. Performance of the vaginal paravaginal repair requires specific expertise to perform it correctly. The long-term effectiveness of paravaginal repair is unknown.

There are no randomized trials that compare outcomes after anterior colporrhaphy versus paravaginal repair. Overall reported rates of anatomical recurrence vary widely from around less than 10% up to 60% [25–27], but subjective improvement and patient satisfaction are achieved in most cases with low reoperation rates [28].

8.4   Posterior Compartment Repair

Gynecologists have routinely performed this surgical approach for over a century, although there is not much evidence regarding its long-term functional and anatomic outcomes. The original description included plication of the pubococcygeus muscles along with plication of the posterior vaginal wall and reconstruction of the perineal body [29].

To date a posterior repair begins with a midline incision extended to the apex of the vagina; the rectovaginal fascia is mobilized from the vaginal epithelium and plicated in the midline with interrupted or continuous absorbable suture. Many authors also describe an anterior plication of the levator ani muscles at this point in the surgery, but it is important to emphasize that this can cause narrowing of the vagina and resultant dyspareunia. Similarly to what has been described for anterior compartment, rectovaginal fascia has to be reattached to the apex and to perineal body.

Although retrospective and prospective reports of posterior repair demonstrate good objective anatomic results ranging from 78 to 97% and success rates for

Fig. 8.7 Anatomic defects in the rectovaginal septum

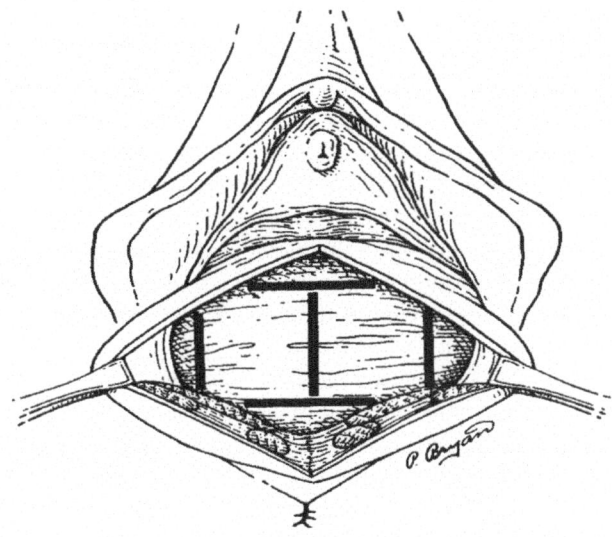

improving defecatory dysfunction in the range of 75%, these same studies report unacceptably high dyspareunia rates ranging from 12 to 27% [30, 31].

However a significant portion of postoperative dyspareunia is likely related to the levator plication, which does not have to be performed in sexually active women.

The site-specific technique is based on the assumption that discrete tears of the rectovaginal septum may result in posterior vaginal wall prolapse. Richardson [32] first published the anatomic sites where tears can occur, and since then this theory has become widely accepted in the urogynecologic community despite a lack of objective supporting evidence. Breaks can be found in the midline, laterally on both sides, and transversally at the apex or at the level of perineal body (Fig. 8.7).

The technique aims for an anatomical repair to close these fascial defects. After the rectovaginal septum is dissected away from the vaginal epithelium, any specific break in the septum is identified, and the defect is repaired with interrupted delayed absorbable sutures. The reported success rates for this procedure range between 82 and 92% with fewer postoperative bothersome symptoms such as dyspareunia, constipation, and defecatory disorders [33, 34].

Abramov et al. [35] in a retrospective comparison of 307 women followed for at least 1 year who underwent standard posterior repair without levator plication or discrete site-specific repair found that site-specific rectocele repair was associated with higher anatomic recurrence rates (11% vs. 4%) and similar rates of dyspareunia and bowel symptoms than standard posterior colporrhaphy.

Perineorrhaphy should be performed with any repair where there is separation of the perineal muscles. This also facilitates the natural posterior deflection of the vagina in the pelvis. After dissection to free the ends of the superficial perineal and bulbocavernosus muscles, they are re-approximated in the midline without tension.

8.4.1 Colpocleisis

In the elderly patient with significant medical problems and sexually inactive, in whom the only alternative is to live with debilitating prolapse, vaginectomy with colpocleisis is a relative short procedure and may be performed without any major complications. Avoiding prolonged surgery with greater dissection and greater risks expedites postoperative recovery. It is unclear whether restoration of anatomy gives advantage to any other functions aside from sexual (i.e., urinary and bowel function). It is also unknown, due to lack of comparative study, whether colpocleisis would be less successful in terms of prolapse cure when compared with sacrospinous fixation or USL suspension.

All colpocleisis surgical techniques involve removal of the vaginal epithelium and subsequently imbricating the vaginal muscularis in apposition to create a tissue septum of support. Numerous variations on this technique, which often vary in the size and amount of epithelium removed, are described [36].

The literature consists mostly of retrospective case series with poorly defined postoperative outcome measures and follow-up. However, success rates after colpocleisis consistently range from 90 to 100% [37–39]. Regret after colpocleisis over loss of coital ability is uncommon ranging from 0 to 12.9%.

References

1. Frick AC, Barber MD, Paraiso MF, Ridgeway B, Jelovsek JE, Walters MD. Attitudes toward hysterectomy in women undergoing evaluation for uterovaginal prolapse. Female Pelvic Med Reconstr Surg. 2013;19:103–9.
2. Gutman R, Maher C. Uterine-preserving POP surgery. Int Urogynecol J. 2013;24:1803–13.
3. Frick AC, Walters MD, Larkin KS, Barber MD. Risk of unanticipated abnormal gynecologic pathology at the time of hysterectomy for uterovaginal prolapse. Am J Obstet Gynecol. 2010;202:507.e1–4.
4. Summers A, Winkel LA, Hussain HK, DeLancey JO. The relationship between anterior and apical compartment support. Am J Obstet Gynecol. 2006;194(5):1438–43.
5. Rooney K, Kenton K, Mueller ER, FitzGerald MP, Brubaker L. Advanced anterior vaginal wall prolapse is highly correlated with apical prolapse. Am J Obstet Gynecol. 2006;195(6):1837–40.
6. McCall CM. Posterior culdoplasty, surgical correction of enterocele during vaginal hysterectomy; a preliminary report. Obstet Gynecol. 1957;10:595–602.
7. Kovac SR, Zimmerman CW. Vaginal hysterectomy. In: Kovac SR, Zimmerman CW, editors. Advances in reconstructive vaginal surgery. Philadelphia: Lippincott Williams & Wilkins; 2007. p. 103–22.
8. Kasturi S, Bentley-Taylor M, Woodman PJ, Terry CL, Hale DS. High uterosacral ligament vaginal vault suspension: comparison of absorbable vs permanent suture for apical fixation. Int Urogynecol J. 2012;23:941–5.
9. Colombo M, Milani R. Sacrospinous ligament fixation and modified McCall culdoplasty during vaginal hysterectomy for advanced uterovaginal prolapse. Am J Obstet Gynecol. 1998;179(1):13–20.
10. Webb MJ, Aronson MP, Ferguson LK, Lee RA. Posthysterectomy vaginal vault prolapse: primary repair in 693 patients. Obstet Gynecol. 1998;92(2):281–5.
11. Spelzini F, Frigerio M, Manodoro S, Interdonato ML, Cesana MC, Verri D, Fumagalli C, Sicuri M, Nicoli E, Polizzi S, Milani R. Modified McCall culdoplasty versus Shull suspension in pelvic prolapse primary repair: a retrospective study. Int Urogynecol J. 2016;28(1):65–71. https://doi.org/10.1007/s00192-016-3016-6.

12. Morgan DM, Rogers AM, Huebner M, Wei JT, DeLancey JO. Heterogeneity in anatomic outcome of sacrospinous ligament fixation for prolapse. Obstet Gynecol. 2007;109: 1424–33.
13. Barber MD, Maher C. Apical prolapse. Int Urogynecol J. 2013;24:1815–33.
14. Matthew D, Barber MD, Brubaker L, Burgio KL. Factorial comparison of two transvaginal surgical approaches and of perioperative behavioral therapy for women with apical vaginal prolapse: the OPTIMAL Randomized Trial. JAMA. 2014;311(10):1023–34.
15. Petri E, Ashok K. Sacrospinous vaginal fixation-current status. Acta Obstet Gynecol Scand. 2011;90:429–36.
16. Maher CF, Murray CJ, Carey MP, et al. Iliococcygeus or sacrospinous fixation for vaginal vault prolapse. Obstet Gynecol. 2001;98:40–4.
17. Serati M, Braga A, Bogani G, Roberti Maggiore UL, Sorice P, Ghezzi F, Salvatore S. Iliococcygeus fixation for the treatment of apical vaginal prolapse: efficacy and safety at 5 years of follow-up. Int Urogynecol J. 2015;26:1007–12.
18. Milani R, Cesana MC, Spelzini F, Sicuri M, Manodoro S, Fruscio R. Iliococcygeus fixation or abdominal sacral colpopexy for the treatment of vaginal vault prolapse: a retrospective cohort study. Int Urogynecol J. 2014;25:279–84.
19. Shull BL, Bachofen C, Coates KW, Kuehl TJ. A transvaginal approach to repair of apical and other associated sites of pelvic organ prolapse with uterosacral ligaments. Am J Obstet Gynecol. 2000;183:1365–73. discussion 1373–1364.
20. Karram M, Goldwasser S, Kleeman S, Steele A, Vassallo B, Walsh P. High uterosacral vaginal vault suspension with fascial reconstruction for vaginal repair of enterocele and vaginal vault prolapse. Am J Obstet Gynecol. 2001;185:1339–43.
21. Silva WA, Pauls RN, Segal JL, Rooney CM, Kleeman SD, Karram MM. Uterosacral ligament vault suspension: five-year outcomes. Obstet Gynecol. 2006;108:255–63.
22. Milani R, Frigerio M, Manodoro S, Cola A, Spelzini F. Transvaginal uterosacral ligament hysteropexy: a retrospective feasibility study. Int Urogynecol J. 2016;28(1):73–6. https://doi.org/10.1007/s00192-016-3036-2.
23. Weber AM, Walters MD. Anterior vaginal prolapse: review of anatomy and techniques of surgical repair. Obstet Gynecol. 1997;89:311–8.
24. Richardson AC, Lyon JB, Williams NL. A new look at pelvic relaxation. Am J Obstet Gynecol. 1976;26:568–73.
25. Porges RF, Smilen SW. Long-term analysis of the surgical management of pelvic support defects. Am J Obstet Gynecol. 1994;171:1518–26.
26. Weber AM, Walters MD, Piedmonte MA, Ballard LA. Anterior colporrhaphy: a randomized trial of three surgical techniques. Am J Obstet Gynecol. 2001;185:1299–306.
27. Shull BL, Benn SJ, Kuehl TJ. Surgical management of prolapse of the anterior vaginal segment: an analysis of support defects, operative morbidity, and anatomic outcome. Am J Obstet Gynecol. 1994;171:1429–36. discussion 1436–1439.
28. Jonsson Funk M, Visco AG, Weidner AC, Pate V, Wu JM. Long-term outcomes of vaginal mesh versus native tissue repair for anterior vaginal wall prolapse. Int Urogynecol J. 2013;(8):1279–85.
29. Jeffcoate TN. Posterior colpoperineorrhaphy. Am J Obstet Gynecol. 1959;77:490–502.
30. Kahn MA, Stanton SL. Posterior colporrhaphy: its effect on bowel and sexual function. Br J Obstet Gynaecol. 1997;104:82–6.
31. Mellegren A, Anzen B, Nilsson BY, Johansson C, Dolk A, Gillgren P, Bremmer S, Holmström B. Results of rectocele repair: a prospective study. Dis Colon Rectum. 1995;38:7–13.
32. Richardson CA. The rectovaginal septum revisited. Its relationship to rectocele and its importance to rectocele repair. Clin Obstet Gynecol. 1993;36:976–83.
33. Cundiff GW, Weidner AC, Visco AG, Addison WA, Bump RC. An anatomic and functional assessment of the discrete defect rectocele repair. Am J Obstet Gynecol. 1998;179:1451–7.
34. Porter WE, Steele A, Walsh P, Kohli N, Karram MM. The anatomic and functional outcomes of defect-specific rectocele repairs. Am J Obstet Gynecol. 1999;181:1353–9.
35. Abramov Y, Gandhi S, Goldberg RP, Botros SM, Kwon C, Sand PK. Site-specific rectocele repair compared with standard posterior colporrhaphy. Obstet Gynecol. 2005;105:314–8.

36. Reiffenstuhl G, Platzer W, Knapstein P. Surgical technique: colpocleisis. In: Vaginal opera-
    tions: surgical anatomy and technique. 2nd ed. Baltimore: Williams and Wilkins; 1996.
    p. 161–76.
37. DeLancey JOL, Morley GW. Total colpocleisis for vaginal eversion. Am J Obstet Gynecol.
    1997;176:1228–35. discussion 1232–1235.
38. Hoffman MS, Cardosi RJ, Lockhart J. Vaginectomy with pelvic herniorrhaphy for prolapse.
    Am J Obstet Gynecol. 2003;189:364–70. discussion 370–371.
39. FitzGerald MP, Brubaker L. Colpocleisis and urinary incontinence. Am J Obstet Gynecol.
    2003;189:1241–4.

Sacrocolpopexy: Conventional Laparoscopic Versus Robot-Assisted Approach

9

Andrea Minervini, Giampaolo Siena, Riccardo Campi, Christian Wagner, Gianni Vittori, Filippo Annino, and Richard Gaston

9.1 Indications to Sacrocolpopexy

Pelvic organ prolapse (POP) is a condition in which the pelvic organs (uterus, bladder and bowel) protrude into or past the vaginal introitus. POP is common and is seen on examination in 40–60% of parous women [1, 2]. Between 6 and 20% of women will have undergone a surgical correction for POP by the age of 80 [3].

The aetiology of POP is complex and multifactorial. Elderly women show a growing incidence, since obesity, smoking women, rising age of the now ageing "baby boom generation" and other risk factors are getting more and more common within the general population.

Treatment of prolapse depends on the severity of the prolapse, its symptoms, the woman's general health and surgeon preference and capabilities. Generally, conservative or mechanical treatments are considered for women with a mild degree of prolapse, those who wish to have more children, the frail or those women unwilling to undergo surgery [4].

For minor prolapses, physical therapy and pelvic floor muscle exercises can be a sufficient form of therapy. In greater degrees of prolapse, a vaginal pessary can be inserted. However, due to the discomfort of endovaginal devices, surgical

A. Minervini, M.D., Ph.D. (✉) · G. Siena, M.D., Ph.D. · R. Campi, M.D. · G. Vittori, M.D., Ph.D.
Department of Urology, University of Florence, Careggi Hospital, Florence, Italy
e-mail: andrea.minervini@unifi.it

C. Wagner, M.D. · R. Gaston, M.D.
Department of Urology, Clinique Saint Augustin, Bordeaux, France

F. Annino, M.D.
Department of Urology, San Donato Hospital Arezzo—Usl Toscana SudEst, Arezzo, Italy

© Springer International Publishing AG, part of Springer Nature 2018　　　　107
V. Li Marzi, M. Serati (eds.), *Management of Pelvic Organ Prolapse*,
Urodynamics, Neurourology and Pelvic Floor Dysfunctions,
https://doi.org/10.1007/978-3-319-59195-7_9

repair is often advised. The annual incidence for POP surgery is stated to be between 1.5 and 1.8 cases per 1000 women-years with the incidence peaking in women between 60 and 69 years [5, 6]. It has also been shown that almost one third of those women undergoing surgery for POP by the age of 80 will require a second surgery thereafter [7].

The aims of surgery for POP repair include restoration of normal vaginal anatomy, restoration or maintenance of normal bladder function, restoration or maintenance of normal bowel function and restoration or maintenance of normal sexual function [4]. Different techniques of surgical repair have been subject to discussion in the last decades.

Sacrocolpopexy (SC) is a well-established and accepted procedure for the treatment of Level 1 POP, i.e. relaxation of sacrouterine ligaments and paracolpium with or without genital prolapse, showing excellent cure rates [8–12]. As such, sacrocolpopexy represents a grade A recommendation procedure for vaginal vault prolapse (VVP) [11]. Further indications include multicompartment POP and recurrent prolapse after failed vaginal repair. For younger (<60 years old) and sexually active women with symptomatic POP, SC with mesh provides anatomic pelvic restoration, durable results and less dyspareunia by maintaining vaginal length and axis and allowing for aseptic mesh placement, thus reducing the risk of mesh infection and erosion.

SC can be performed laparoscopically with or without robotic assistance. At present, laparoscopic SC (LSC) is widely adopted and there are many reports showing durable results [13]. However, indications and technical aspects are not standardized and vary from country to country. Moreover, the technique is considered challenging because of the multiple sutures required. Robotic technology has been marketed based on several possible advantages, including better visualization, extreme manoeuvrability resulting in easy sutures and greater efficiency. Therefore, the use of robotic SC (RASC) in the management of female POP appears to be increasing [14].

9.2   Surgical Technique

9.2.1   Robot-Assisted Sacrocolpopexy (RASC)

9.2.1.1 Patient Positioning

The patient is placed in a supine position on a padded vacuum mattress, with legs abducted on Allen's stirrups to help positioning the da Vinci robot. Once the patient is positioned in Trendelenburg position, the perineum should be at the edge of the operating bed to facilitate the use of the vaginal manipulator or of the malleable vaginal retractor. Antibiotic prophylaxis is administered during the induction of the anaesthesia. A Foley catheter is inserted once the surgical field has been prepared.

The operating bed must provide a Trendelenburg position, and in case of a planned contemporary stress incontinence surgery, the legs of the patient should be

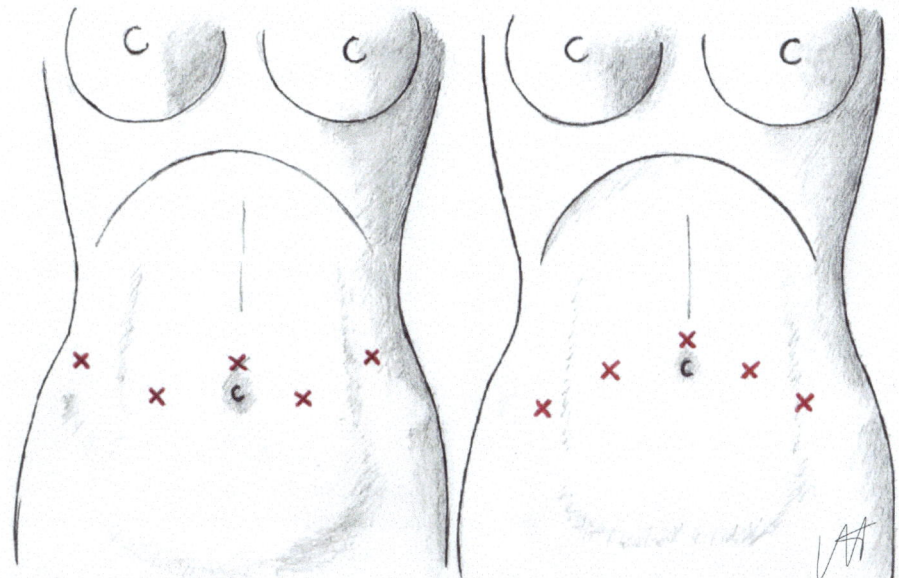

Fig. 9.1 Port placement for robot-assisted sacrocolpopexy (RASC). "W"-shaped (left) and "linear"-shaped (right) port configurations

movable to a lithotomic position at the end of the procedure; otherwise the patient should be repositioned and the surgical field redone.

9.2.1.2 Port Placement

The ports are placed in a "W"-shaped configuration (Fig. 9.1, left) or in a "linear" configuration (Fig. 9.1, right) as for pelvic floor surgery, i.e. robot-assisted laparoscopic prostatectomy. The camera trocar can be placed at the level of the umbilicus. The operating table is positioned into a moderate Trendelenburg position around 20°–25° head down, helping to keep the intestine away from the surgical field.

Four robotic arms are generally used, utilizing the camera (with a 0° or a 30° down scope). The robotic instruments employed for the procedure include one Maryland bipolar forceps, a fenestrated grasper (ProGrasp or Cadiere forceps), robotic monopolar curved scissors (Hot Shears scissors) and one large needle driver. Furthermore, a vaginal manipulator or a malleable vaginal retractor is used to manipulate the vagina during the procedure.

9.2.1.3 Mesh Configuration

A non-absorbable (polypropylene or soft Prolene), 15 × 10 cm wide mesh is normally used, and it is advisable to have it prepared beforehand.

The mesh is cut into two pieces: the anterior and the posterior mesh. The posterior mesh is 4 cm wide × 6 cm long with a plate that corresponds to the isolated rectovaginal space, with a concave profile at the tip and two sutures 10–12 cm long with a 2 cm tail ligated at the two lateral edges of the concave tip and with a central

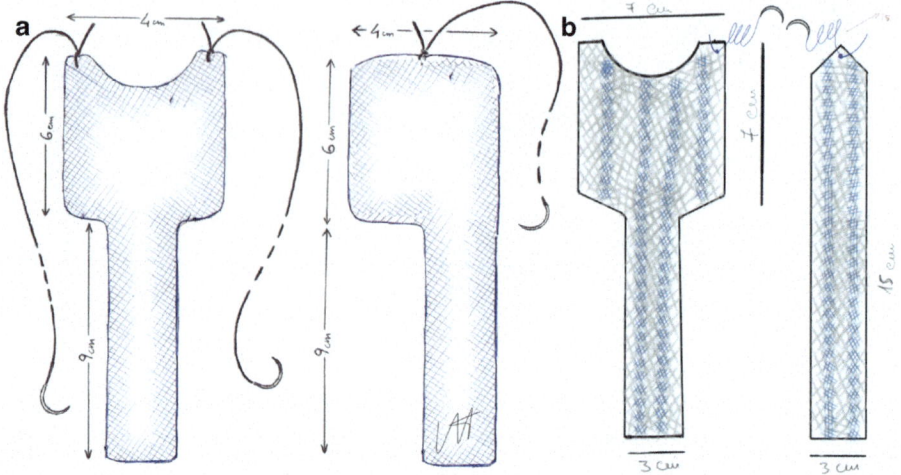

Fig. 9.2 Posterior and anterior mesh configuration. (**a**) Posterior (*left*) and Anterior (*right*) mesh configuration used at the Department of Urology of Careggi Hospital in Florence (Italy). (**b**) Posterior (*left*) and Anterior (*right*) mesh configuration used at the Departments of Urology of San Donato Hospital in Arezzo (Italy) and of the Clinique Saint-Augustin de Bordeaux (France)

tail (Fig. 9.2a, left). The anterior mesh is 4 cm wide × 6 cm long, with a plate that corresponds to the isolated anterior vaginal wall, with a convex tip and one or two 16 cm long non-absorbable plurifilament sutures with a 2 cm tail ligated at the very tip concave edges and with a lateral right-sided tail (Fig. 9.2a, right). Another possible mesh configuration is shown in Fig. 9.2b. The total length of both meshes should be approximately 15 cm; any extra length of the tails is of no importance.

9.2.1.4 Promontory Exposure and Posterior Dissection

After port placement and docking of the robot, the right iliac vessels and right ureter, the uterus along with right ovary and tube, the vaginal stump, the Douglas pouch and the rectum are identified as the most important landmarks (Fig. 9.3). If present, to gain a better exposure of the Douglas pouch, the uterus is lifted upwards with either a transcutaneous nylon 0 or 2–0 stitch or with a uterine manipulator. Alternatively, to have a dynamic exposition and traction, a ProGrasp forceps can be used.

The peritoneum that overlays the promontory is then incised on the right side of the sigmoid colon; care is taken to avoid damage to the iliac vessels and the right ureter. Once the peritoneum is opened, the sacrum and the anterior longitudinal ligament are identified. The peritoneal incision is extended caudally till the Douglas pouch on the right side following and crossing the right uterosacral ligament (Fig. 9.3). The posterior vaginal wall is mobilized upwards by the vaginal valve and dissected off the rectum by opening the rectovaginal Douglas space (Fig. 9.4). The malleable vaginal retractor inserted in the posterior vaginal wall cul-de-sac should be anteverted as much as possible to stretch the uterosacral ligaments. At this stage,

Fig. 9.3 Incision of the peritoneum. Superficial incision of the peritoneum overlaying the promontory, extended caudally till the Douglas pouch on the right side, taking care to avoid damage to the iliac vessels and the right ureter

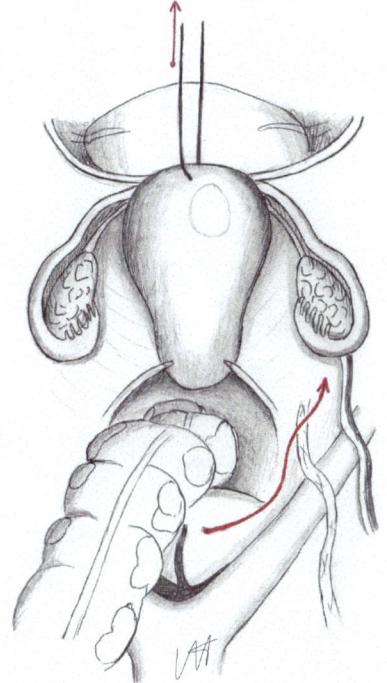

leaving a bridge of peritoneum between the posterior peritoneal incision and the Douglas opening might facilitate the peritoneal closure and enable the surgeons to close the Douglas pouch immediately after the posterior mesh fixation, thus not having to suspend it again later for peritoneal closure.

The inferior layer of the peritoneum is pulled downward to access to the avascular plane of the rectovaginal fascia. Dissection should start medially, close to the posterior vaginal wall.

The dissection should be carried out bluntly through the perirectal fat until the levator ani aponeurosis is prepared bilaterally. At this stage, care should be taken not to damage the rectal vascularization (haemorrhoidal plexus) (Fig. 9.4).

9.2.1.5 Posterior Mesh Fixation and Douglas Closure
The pre-fashioned posterior mesh is suture-fixated with a braided non-reabsorbable suture at the dorsal, most distal part of the mobilized posterior vaginal wall and posterolaterally to the distal levator ani aponeurosis without taking the muscle fibres within the suture to avoid trapping the levator ani fibres (Fig. 9.5). At this stage, the external preparation of a posterior mesh that incorporates the two sutures can speed up this surgical step.

Lateral injury to the middle rectal artery and rectal nerve plexus must be avoided at this level. Therefore, a minimal dissection at the level of the rectum is recommended to reduce the incidence of postoperative constipation. A rectocele can make this step of the procedure more challenging.

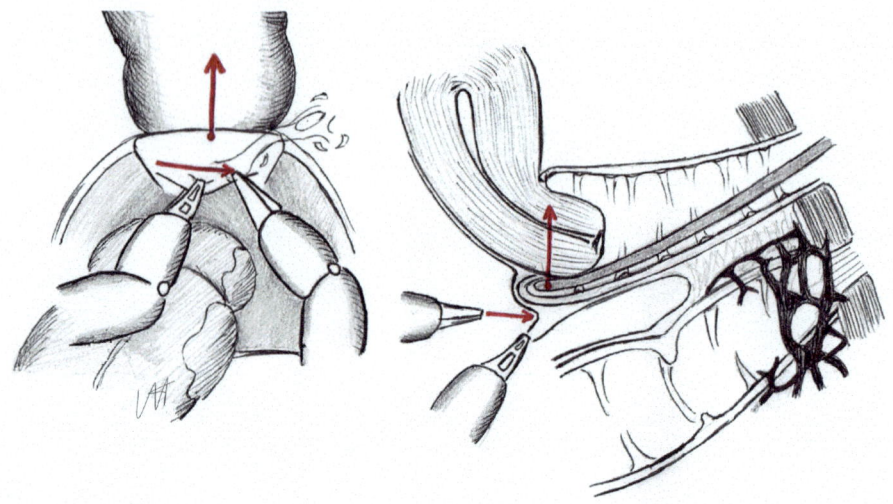

Fig. 9.4 Valve insertion. The malleable vaginal valve is inserted in the posterior vaginal cul-de-sac to mobilize upwards the uterus and the posterior vaginal wall. The rectovaginal Douglas space is opened and the posterior vaginal wall is dissected off the rectum

Fig. 9.5 Posterior mesh fixation. The pre-fashioned posterior mesh is fixated with a non-reabsorbable suture to the distal levator ani aponeurosis. A solid but superficial suture must be made to avoid including the muscle fibres within the suture and trapping them

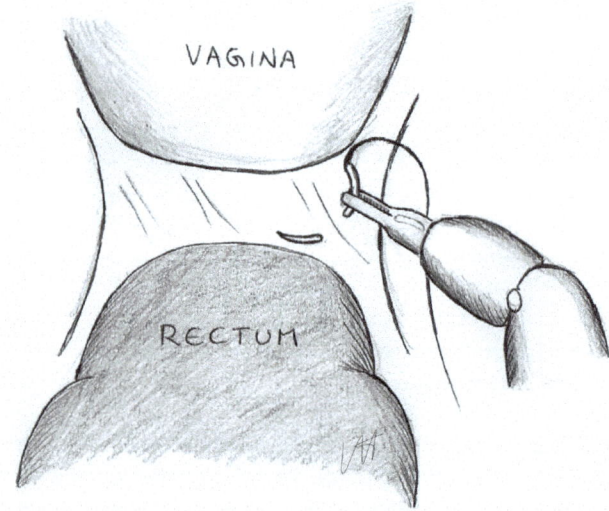

At this moment, the peritoneal breach at the level of the Douglas pouch can be closed with a 3–0 braided absorbable suture and the tail of the posterior mesh left extraperitoneally passing behind the bridge of the peritoneum left between the posterior peritoneal incision and the Douglas.

9.2.1.6 Vesico-Vaginal Dissection

In an analogue fashion, the peritoneum between the bladder and vagina is then incised to mobilize the anterior vaginal wall. The vaginal retractor is inserted in the anterior fornix and pushed downward (Fig. 9.6). Dissection starts at the midline

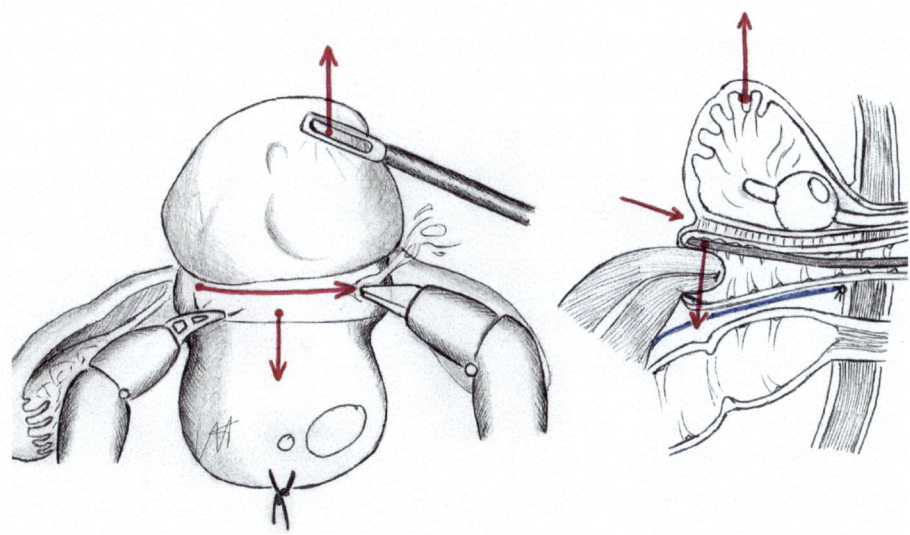

Fig. 9.6 Vesico-vaginal dissection. The vaginal retractor is inserted in the anterior fornix and pushed downward. The bladder is gently lifted upwards by the assisted or the robotic third arm. The peritoneum between the bladder and the vagina is then incised to mobilize the anterior vaginal wall. Dissection begins at the midline between the vagina and the bladder. The white pearl surface of the anterior vaginal wall is a landmark point

between the bladder and vagina. The white pearl surface of the anterior vaginal wall is a landmark point. Bipolar or monopolar haemostatic control of small perivaginal vascular structures is sometimes necessary. The vaginal valve should be inserted with enough tension to provide the right exposure of the dorsal vaginal wall to help finding the correct plane between the bladder and the anterior vaginal wall (Fig. 9.6). Dissection should be carried out laterally to expose the anterolateral vaginal wall and distally until the retrotrigonal area is reached. To identify this limit is possible to move the Foley balloon. At this level it is important not to proceed too distally towards the posterior bladder neck to reduce the incidence of urgency.

9.2.1.7 Anterior Mesh Fixation

The anterior mesh can be now fixed on both sides of the dorsal vaginal stump with a 2–0 braided non-reasorbable running sutures (Fig. 9.7). Attention should be used to stay superficial on the vaginal wall avoiding the needle to pass through. Also for the anterior mesh placement, the external mesh preparation can speed up this surgical step.

In case of a still existing uterus, the tail of the anterior mesh is brought cranially to the promontory through a tunnelled perforation of the right broad ligament (Fig. 9.7). In these cases, a further single or double 2–0 braided stitch can be placed to fix the mesh anteriorly to the cervix of the uterus to stabilize it and avoid a late down sliding.

9.2.1.8 POP Correction and Mesh Fixation to the Sacral Promontory

The sigmoid colon is then again retracted to expose the promontory. If needed, a further load could be done at this time on the vaginal valve to correct the POP. The

Fig. 9.7 Anterior mesh fixation. The anterior mesh can be now fixed on both sides of the dorsal vaginal stump with non-reabsorbable running sutures. Attention should be used to stay superficial on the vaginal wall avoiding the needle to pass through. The tail of the anterior mesh is brought cranially to the promontory through a tunnelled perforation of the right broad ligament

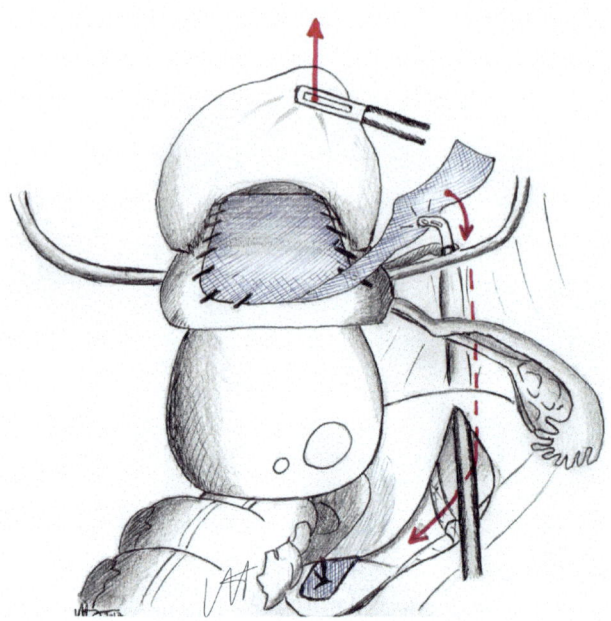

tails of both meshes are unrolled and put under only slight to moderate tension. The mesh is then fixated with one or two non-absorbable, 0 plurifilament interrupted sutures at the longitudinal ligament of the promontory bone. At this moment, the vaginal manipulator is extracted from the vagina to verify the result of the POP correction.

9.2.1.9 Reperitonealization

Finally, the mesh is completely retroperitonealized. It is very important to reach a complete peritoneal cover over the mesh in order to avoid future bowel herniation, obstruction, adhesions or inflammatory responses. A drain is usually unnecessary.

9.2.1.10 Postoperative Course

The transurethral Foley catheter can be removed the next morning. A vaginal oestrogen ointment starting 6 weeks prior to surgery can be further administered for another 3 months at least. After restoring the correct anatomy, a hidden stress urinary incontinence may become evident. In this case, an implant of a tension-free tape after 3–6 months can be done.

9.2.2 Laparoscopic Sacrocolpopexy (LSC)

The laparoscopic and robotic approaches share most of the surgical steps. However there are some differences of the laparoscopic procedure. As the fourth robotic arm is lacking, tractions can be either done by the assistant or by sutures placed ad hoc.

Haptic feedback can be of help to underline the promontory especially in obese patients and to apply the correct tension on the meshes especially on the anterior mesh. During the laparoscopic procedure, it is also possible to modulate Trendelenburg according to the different steps of the procedure without overloading the patient with a severe head down position throughout the procedure.

The first surgeon is on the left and the assistant on the right side. A second assistant uses the vaginal manipulator or the malleable retractor and sits between the legs of the patient. The scrub nurse is on the left side of the surgeon and the instruments table is on her/his left.

Four trocars are usually necessary. Main landmarks are umbilicus, symphysis and right and left anterior superior iliac crests. A 12 mm or Hasson trocar is positioned intraumbilically for the 0° or 30° camera, another 5 mm trocar is placed halfway between the umbilicus and the pubic symphysis, and two 5 mm trocars (or one 5 mm and one 12 mm trocar) are placed 2–3 cm medially to the anterior superior iliac crest on both sides. The required instruments are atraumatic graspers, bipolar forceps, monopolar curved scissors, suction device, two laparoscopic needle drivers (alternatively one laparoscopic needle driver and one Maryland forceps) and harmonic scalpel (optional).

Once the trocars are inserted and the pneumoperitoneum induced, the procedure starts by mobilizing the sigmoid colon to expose the rectouterine pouch. The sigmoid colon can be fixated to the abdominal wall on the left side by a suture, and, if present, the uterus is lifted upwards with either a transcutaneous 0 or 2–0 stitch with straight needle or with a uterine manipulator.

During the rectovaginal dissection, to expose the anterolateral surface of the rectum, the posterior vaginal wall and the levator ani aponeurosis, the orientation of the 30° scope can be positioned upwards for a better vision of the rectovaginal space.

The mesh is fixed on both sides of the levator ani fascia. The stitch is positioned with a 180° rotation of the needle. The rectouterine pouch is eventually closed, the mesh is extraperitonealized and the uterosacral ligaments are approximated.

The peritoneum overlaying of the promontory is then incised on the right side of the sigmoid colon as during the robotic operation. The promontory is felt with the haptic feedback of the tip of a laparoscopic instrument. The first assistant pulls the intestine backwards with the laparoscopic Johan. The posterior peritoneum is incised with the tip of the monopolar scissors, while the left hand holds a grasper that lifts the peritoneum up to avoid injuries of the presacral vessels.

After anterior vaginal wall dissection and anterior mesh fixation, the sigmoid colon is again retracted laterally to expose the promontory. A further load could be done at this time on the vaginal valve to correct the POP. The tails of both meshes are unrolled and put under only slight to moderate tension. The haptic feedback at this stage can facilitate this surgical step especially if the uterus is still in place; thus its presence makes it not possible to visually verify the restored pelvic anatomy. At this moment, the vaginal retractor or uterine manipulator is extracted from the vagina to verify the result of the POP correction.

9.3   Outcomes and Complications of Abdominal and Minimally Invasive Sacrocolpopexy: Review of the Current Literature

Since its introduction in 1962 [15], sacrocolpopexy has showed effective and durable outcomes for apical prolapse repair. While *open* sacrocolpopexy has represented the standard technique for many years, the advent of minimally invasive surgery (laparoscopic and robotic) has revolutionized the surgical approach becoming the most widely used technique over the last decade.

9.3.1   Sacrocolpopexy Vs. Vaginal Surgery

A 2016 Cochrane review identified six randomized controlled trials (RCTs) comparing sacrocolpopexy to vaginal prolapse repair [16]. This systematic review included three trials comparing *abdominal* sacrocolpopexy (ASC) to sacrospinous ligament suspension (SSLS) [17–19], one trial comparing ASC to uterosacral ligament suspension (USLS) [20], one trial comparing laparoscopic sacrocolpopexy (LSC) to transvaginal mesh repair [21] and one trial comparing abdominal or laparoscopic sacrocolpopexy to uterosacral ligament suspension (USLS) with mesh augmentation [16]. This meta-analysis concluded that vaginal surgery (including a broad spectrum of surgical techniques) with and without mesh placement was associated with worse postoperative outcomes as compared to sacrocolpopexy and, in particular, with higher risk of awareness of prolapse (RR 2.11; 95% CI 1.1–4.2), recurrent prolapse (RR 1.9; 95% CI 1.3–2.7), repeat prolapse surgery (RR 2.3; 95% CI 1.2–4.3), postoperative SUI (RR 1.9; 95% CI 1.2–2.9) and dyspareunia (RR 2.5; 95% 1.2–5.5) [16, 22].

Improved anatomic outcomes after sacrocolpopexy compared with native tissue (non-mesh) vaginal repair surgery were also confirmed by another systematic review of the literature performed by the Society of Gynecologic Surgeons Systematic Review Group [23]. However, in this study, that comprised both randomized trials and cohort studies; no difference was found between reoperation rates and postoperative sexual function among the two groups. In this review, sacrocolpopexy was found to be associated with higher rates of ileus or small bowel obstruction (2.7% vs. 0.2%, $p < 0.01$), mesh or suture complications (4.2% vs. 0.4%, $p < 0.01$) and thromboembolic disease (0.6% vs. 0.1%, $p = 0.03$).

9.3.2   Abdominal Sacrocolpopexy (ASC)

Abdominal sacrocolpopexy (ASC) has been shown to be a highly effective procedure for the repair of apical prolapse by several observational studies and clinical trials, with a success rate ranging from 78 to 100% [22]. Many trials demonstrated optimal outcomes in terms of symptoms, urinary function and quality of life after ASC for POP [18, 24].

A systematic review of the literature on ASC reported median rates of reoperation for POP recurrence, postoperative stress urinary incontinence and mesh erosion of 4.4% (range 0–18.2%), 4.9% (range 1.2–30.9%) and 3.4%, respectively [25].

Although the definition of success after sacrocolpopexy is still variable across the published series, the long-term follow-up (5–7 years) date from the CARE trial (E-CARE) demonstrated objective failure rates after ASC of 24–48% and a cumulative mesh erosion rate of 10.5% by 7 years [26].

With regard to surgical complications, the systematic review of the literature by Nygaard et al. showed that the most frequently reported complications after ASC are, beyond mesh erosion, wound complications (occurring in 4.6% of patients), bleeding (in 4.4% of patients), cystotomy (in 3.1% of patients), ureteral injury (in 1.0% of patients), bowel injury (in 1.6% of patients) and incisional hernias (in 5% of patients) [25]. Gastrointestinal morbidity was found to be a significant adverse event after ASC in 1 of 20 women in the CARE trial [27].

9.3.3 Laparoscopic and Robotic Sacrocolpopexy

Standard laparoscopic sacrocolpopexy (LSC) technique has been described for years since it minimizes the surgical trauma of the open approach, while providing comparable success rate. However, suturing and mesh handling result more challenging and time-consuming, representing a limitation to a wider adoption of the laparoscopic approach. Most RCTs showed that LSC is as effective as open ASC with the advantages of reduced rates of intraoperative bleeding, hospitalization and wound complications [22, 28, 29].

LSC has therefore been used by many surgeons worldwide over the last decade as a minimally invasive alternative to ASC with the aim to reproduce the surgical principles of open surgery while reducing perioperative morbidity and length of hospitalization associated with standard laparotomy. To date, several prospective and retrospective series have demonstrated good short- and mid-term success rates of LSC with mean objective and subjective success rates of 60–100% and 79–98%, respectively [30–32]. Accordingly, LSC has been shown to achieve significant improvements in subjective symptoms and quality of life in several prospective series [33, 34].

Despite the clinical advantages of LSC, adoption of this approach worldwide is limited by the steep learning curve and the challenging technical aspects of the procedure, mainly related to laparoscopic suturing and knot-tying skills that are required for mesh fixation. In a study evaluating the learning curve of LSC in the first 206 cases performed by a single surgeon, operative time reached a steady state of 175 min after 90 cases; the authors concluded that *adequate* learning of the procedure (defined according to a careful evaluation of operative times and complication rates) required 60 cases [35].

Since the growing availability of the da Vinci® surgical robotic system, more and more complex laparoscopic reconstructive procedures have been translated into a robot-assisted approach, such as Anderson-Hynes pyeloplasty or ureteral reimplantation. Indeed, the da Vinci system offers the technical advantages of 3D vision, up to tenfold magnification and unprecedented freedom of movement of the robotic instruments, including an intuitive motion of the surgeon's hands to steer the instruments. This combination of advantages enables surgeons with little experience in standard laparoscopy to switch to a robot-assisted laparo-scopic approach and experienced laparoscopic surgeons to unlimited surgical abilities.

The first RASC was described by Di Marco and colleagues in 2004 [36]; since then, it has gained more and more popularity among urologists and gynaecologists.

The increased number of robotic sacrocolpopexies performed worldwide may reflect the need to overcome the relatively long learning curve required for LSC. Indeed, many surgeons have turned to the robotic platform to offer patients a minimally invasive approach to sacrocolpopexy, with the aim to facilitate techni-cally challenging steps of the procedure and to shorten the overall learning curve by taking advantage of the improved surgeon's vision, dexterity and ergonomics [22]. Limited data suggest that both operating time and surgical efficiency improve sig-nificantly after 20 RASCs [37].

A recent systematic review of the literature involving 1488 patients undergoing RASC showed objective and subjective cure rates of 84–100% and 92–95%, respec-tively, with mesh erosion rates of 2% (range 0–8%) [8]. Overall, postoperative com-plication rate after RASC in this meta-analysis was 11% (range 0–43%), severe complications being recorded in 2% of patients. Conversion to open ASC occurred in <1% (range 0–5%).

To date, two randomized trials have assessed the outcomes after LSC vs. RASC [33, 38]. The results of the most recent multicentre randomized trial by Anger et al. outline that RASC had higher *initial* and *6-week* hospital costs ($19,616 compared with $11,573 and $20,898 compared with $12,170, respectively, both $P < 0.001$) compared to ASC. However, the 6-week hospital costs did not differ among the two groups after the exclusion of the costs for robot purchase and maintenance ($13,867 compared with $12,170; $P = 0.06$) [38]. Operative time and postoperative 1-week pain scores were higher in the RASC group, while 1-year symptoms, quality of life and sexual outcomes did not differ between the two groups [39]. In the other single-centre randomized trial comparing the outcomes of RASC and LSC in women with stage II–IV post-hysterectomy vaginal prolapse, Paraiso et al. confirmed that both operative time and costs were significantly higher after RASC. Postoperative pain and need of non-steroidal anti-inflammatory medications were also higher in the RASC group, while no differences in anatomical results or quality of life measures were recorded at 1-year follow-up [33].

Beyond the results of these randomized trials, a recent review of several com-parative studies outlined that in the majority of the available series both success and complication rates were similar between LSC and RASC, at a cost of longer opera-tive time for RASC [22].

Complications and sequelae of minimally invasive sacrocolpopexy mainly include de novo stress urinary incontinence, bowel dysfunction (including dysche-zia, obstructed defecation and outlet constipation), dyspareunia, blood loss, conversion to open surgery and mesh erosion. In their meta-analysis, Serati et al. reported a 1% conversion rate from a robot-assisted approach to other approaches. Seventy-nine percent of conversions were from robotic to open surgery, due to technical difficulties related to adhesions, limited exposure and management of complications [8]. Twenty-one percent of conversions were from robotic to laparoscopy, in 14% of the cases due to robot malfunctions and in 7% due to adhesions.

Regarding complications and perioperative adverse events of LSC vs. RASC, a retrospective analysis by Unger et al. showed that bladder injury and estimated blood loss greater than 500 mL resulted higher in the robotic group (3.3% vs. 0.4%, $p = 0.04$, and 2.5% vs. 0%, $p = 0.01$, respectively) [40]. On the contrary, a meta-analysis of six smaller studies found lower blood loss (50 vs. 155 mL, $p < 0.001$) after RASC but similar rates of other complications when compared to LSC [8].

Recurrence and vaginal mesh exposure rates following LSC or hysteropexy were 4–18% (at 12–14 months of follow-up) and 1–7%, respectively [22]. The same authors showed mean rates of reoperation for prolapse recurrence and of de novo stress urinary incontinence after ASC of 2% and 5%, respectively. Mean reoperation rate for LSC has been shown to be 5.6%, with 3.4% of patients experiencing complications.

Vaginal mesh exposure rates were comparable regardless the surgical approach (open, laparoscopic or robotic) [41]. Of note, the risk of vaginal mesh exposure was shown to be significantly higher if concomitant hysterectomy was performed (8.6%), as compared to sacrocolpopexy for post-hysterectomy prolapse (2.2%) ($p < 0.05$) [42].

Visceral (bladder, rectum) mesh exposure has been reported rarely (<0.1%) following sacrocolpopexy or hysteropexy (performed with either open, laparoscopic or robotic approach) [13, 43]. Spondylitis, as well as pelvic abscess, had been reported rarely following LSC, with an estimated prevalence of 0.1–0.2% [22]. Concerning LSC, conversion to open ASC is rarely considered as a complication. However, mean conversion rate is 3%, according to the surgeons' experience [22]. Mean bladder injury rate ranges from 0.6 to 2% during ASC and LSC or RASC. Bladder injury may occur due to trocar placement, tissue dissection or suture placement. Injuries have been managed by immediate repair and extended duration of indwelling catheter. Mean bowel injury rate ranges from 0.07 to 1% [22]. Perioperative blood loss is decreased using LSC when compared to ASC. However, blood loss is limited (150–200 mL), and the requirement of transfusion is rare (<1%), whatever the surgical route. In this regard, concomitant hysterectomy may increase the overall blood loss. Obstructed defecation is rarely reported (2%) following sacrocolpopexy. However, small bowel obstruction and port site hernias have been reported in the literature (0.2%). Finally, vascular injuries represent rare complications (<1%) of sacrocolpopexy. Of note, cases of patient deaths occurring after vaginal surgery or open or laparoscopic sacrocolpopexy/hysteropexy have been described [22]. Concerning abdominal surgery, mortality rates ranged from 0.05 to 0.1%, with no difference found between open and laparoscopic surgical approaches [43].

Conclusion

The surgical outcomes of SC for the treatment of POP are excellent and similar between RASC and LSC. However, RASC is highly expensive and more time-consuming. Though RASC may have other benefits, such as reduction of the learning curve and increased ergonomics or dexterity, these remain to be demonstrated. With the actual excellent surgical results and the future decline of costs, the indication to RASC is expected to grow.

References

1. Handa VL, Garrett E, Hendrix S, et al. Progression and remission of pelvic organ prolapse: a longitudinal study of menopausal women. Am J Obstet Gynecol. 2004;190(1):27–32.
2. Hendrix SL, Clark A, Nygaard I, et al. Pelvic organ prolapse in the Women's Health Initiative: gravity and gravidity. Am J Obstet Gynecol. 2002;186(6):1160–6.
3. Smith FJ, Holman CD, Moorin RE, Tsokos N. Lifetime risk of undergoing surgery for pelvic organ prolapse. Obstet Gynecol. 2010;116(5):1096–100.
4. Maher C, Feiner B, Baessler K, Schmid C. Surgical management of pelvic organ prolapse in women. Cochrane Database Syst Rev. 2013;30(4):CD004014.
5. Boyles SH, Weber AM, Meyn L. Procedures for pelvic organ prolapse in the United States, 1979-1997. Am J Obstet Gynecol. 2003;188(1):108–15.
6. Shah AD, Kohli N, Rajan SS, Hoyte L. The age distribution, rates, and types of surgery for pelvic organ prolapse in the USA. Int Urogynecol J Pelvic Floor Dysfunct. 2008;19(3):421–8.
7. Gerten KA, Markland AD, Lloyd LK, Richter HE. Prolapse and incontinence surgery in older women. J Urol. 2008;179(6):2111–8.
8. Serati M, Bogani G, Sorice P, et al. Robot-assisted sacrocolpopexy for pelvic organ prolapse: a systematic review and meta-analysis of comparative studies. Eur Urol. 2014;66(2):303–18.
9. Pan K, Zhang Y, Wang Y, et al. A systematic review and meta-analysis of conventional laparoscopic sacrocolpopexy versus robot-assisted laparoscopic sacrocolpopexy. Int J Gynaecol Obstet. 2016;132(3):284–91.
10. Ploumidis A, Spinoit AF, De Naeyer G, et al. Robot-assisted sacrocolpopexy for pelvic organ prolapse: surgical technique and outcomes at a single high-volume institution. Eur Urol. 2014;65(1):138–45.
11. Merseburger AS, Herrmann TR, Shariat SF, et al. EAU guidelines on robotic and single-site surgery in urology. Eur Urol. 2013;64(2):277–91.
12. Costantini E, Brubaker L, Cervigni M, et al. Sacrocolpopexy for pelvic organ prolapse: evidence-based review and recommendations. Eur J Obstet Gynecol Reprod Biol. 2016;205:60–5.
13. Lee RK, Mottrie A, Payne CK, Waltregny D. A review of the current status of laparoscopic and robot-assisted sacrocolpopexy for pelvic organ prolapse. Eur Urol. 2014;65(6):1128–37.
14. Clifton MM, Pizarro-Berdichevsky J, Goldman HB. Robotic female pelvic floor reconstruction: a review. Urology. 2016;91:33–40.
15. Lane F. Repair of posthysterectomy vaginal-vault prolapse. Obstet Gynecol. 1962;20:72–7.
16. Maher C, Feiner B, Baessler K, et al. Surgery for women with apical vaginal prolapse. Cochrane Database Syst Rev. 2016; (10).
17. Benson JT, Lucente V, McClellan E. Vaginal versus abdominal reconstructive surgery for the treatment of pelvic support defects: a prospective randomized study with long-term outcome evaluation. Am J Obstet Gynecol. 1996;175(6):1418–21.
18. Maher CF, Qatawneh A, Dwyer P, et al. Abdominal sacral colpopexy or vaginal sacrospinous colpopexy for vaginal vault prolapse. A prospective randomized trial. Am J Obstet Gynecol. 2004;190:20–6.

19. Lo TS, Wang AC. Abdominal colposacropexy and sacrospinous ligament suspension for severe uterovaginal prolapse: a comparison. J Gynecol Surg. 1998;14:59–64.
20. Rondini C, Braun H, Alvarez J, et al. High uterosacral vault suspension vs sacrocolpopexy for treating apical defects: a randomized controlled trial with twelve months follow-up. Int Urogynecol J. 2015;26(8):1131–8.
21. Maher C, Feiner B, DeCuyper E, et al. Laparoscopic sacral colpopexy versus total vaginal mesh for vaginal vault prolapse: a randomized trial. Am J Obstet Gynecol. 2011;204(4):360 e1–7.
22. Abrams P, Cardozo L, Wagg A, Wein A. Incontinence. 6th edition 2017. 6th International Consultation on Incontinence. Tokyo: ICS-ICUD; 2016. ISBN: 978-0-9569607-3-3.
23. Siddiqui NY, Grimes CL, Casiano ER, et al. Mesh sacrocolpopexy compared with native tissue vaginal repair: a systematic review and meta-analysis. Obstet Gynecol. 2015;125(1):44–55.
24. Brubaker L, Nygaard I, Richter HE, et al. Two-year outcomes after sacrocolpopexy with and without burch to prevent stress urinary incontinence. Obstet Gynecol. 2008;112:49–55.
25. Nygaard IE, McCreery R, Brubaker L, et al. Abdominal sacrocolpopexy: a comprehensive review. Obstet Gynecol. 2004;104(4):805–23.
26. Nygaard I, Brubaker L, Zyczynski HM, et al. Long-term outcomes following abdominal sacrocolpopexy for pelvic organ prolapse. JAMA. 2013;309(19):2016–24.
27. Whitehead WE, Bradley CS, Brown MB, et al. Gastrointestinal complications following abdominal sacrocolpopexy for advanced pelvic organ prolapse. Am J Obstet Gynecol. 2007;197:78 e1–7.
28. Freeman R, Pantazis K, Thomson A, et al. A randomised controlled trial of abdominal versus laparoscopic sacrocolpopexy for the treatment of post-hysterectomy vaginal vault prolapse: LAS study. Int Urogynecol J. 2013;24:377–84.
29. Tyson MD, Wolter CE. A comparison of 30-day surgical outcomes for minimally invasive and open sacrocolpopexy. Neurourol Urodyn. 2015;34(2):151–5.
30. Higgs PJ, Chua HL, Smith AR. Long term review of laparoscopic sacrocolpopexy. BJOG. 2005;112(8):1134–8.
31. Rivoire C, Botchorishvili R, Canis M, et al. Complete laparoscopic treatment of genital prolapse with meshes including vaginal promontofixation and anterior repair: a series of 138 patients. J Minim Invasive Gynecol. 2007;14(6):712–8.
32. Sarlos D, Brandner S, Kots L, et al. Laparoscopic sacrocolpopexy for uterine and post-hysterectomy prolapse: anatomical results, quality of life and perioperative outcome—a prospective study with 101 cases. Int Urogynecol J Pelvic Floor Dysfunct. 2008;19(10):1415–22.
33. Paraiso M, Jelovsek J, Frick A, Chen C, Barber M. Laparoscopic compared with robotic sacrocolpopexy for vaginal prolapse: a randomized controlled trial. Obstet Gynecol. 2011;118(5):1005–13.
34. Sergent F, Resch B, Loisel C, Bisson V, Schaal JP, Marpeau L. Mid-term outcome of laparoscopic sacrocolpopexy with anterior and posterior polyester mesh for treatment of genitourinary prolapse. Eur J Obstet Gynecol Reprod Biol. 2011;156:217–22.
35. Claerhout F, Roovers JP, Lewi P, et al. Implementation of laparoscopic sacrocolpopexy—a single centre's experience. Int Urogynecol J Pelvic Floor Dysfunct. 2009;20(9):1119–25.
36. Di Marco DS, Chow GK, Gettman MT, Elliott DS. Robotic-assisted laparoscopic sacrocolpopexy for treatment of vaginal vault prolapse. Urology. 2004;63(2):373–6.
37. Geller EJ, Lin FC, Matthews CA. Analysis of robotic performance times to improve operative efficiency. J Minim Invasive Gynecol. 2013;20(1):43–8.
38. Anger J, Mueller E, Tarnay C, Smith B, Stroupe K, Rosenman A, et al. Robotic compared with laparoscopic sacrocolpopexy: a randomized controlled trial. Obstet Gynecol. 2014;123(1):5–12.
39. Mueller MG, Jacobs KM, Mueller ER, et al. Outcomes in 450 women after minimally invasive abdominal sacrocolpopexy for pelvic organ prolapse. Female Pelvic Med Reconstr Surg. 2016;22(4):267–71.

40. Unger CA, Walters MD, Ridgeway B, et al. Incidence of adverse events after uterosacral colpopexy for uterovaginal and posthysterectomy vault prolapse. Am J Obstet Gynecol. 2015;212(5):603.e1–7.
41. De Gouveia De Sa M, Claydon LS, Whitlow B, Dolcet Artahona MA. Robotic versus laparoscopic sacrocolpopexy for treatment of prolapse of the apical segment of the vagina: a systematic review and meta-analysis. Int Urogynecol J. 2016;27(3):355–66.
42. Gutman R, Maher C. Uterine-preserving prolapse surgery. Int Urogynecol J. 2013;24(11):1803–13.
43. De Gouveia De Sa M, Claydon LS, Whitlow B, Dolcet Artahona MA. Laparoscopic versus open sacrocolpopexy for treatment of prolapse of the apical segment of the vagina: a systematic review and meta-analysis. Int Urogynecol J. 2016;27(1):3–17.

Transvaginal Mesh Repair for Pelvic Organ Prolapse: Toward a New Era

10

Vincenzo Li Marzi, Jacopo Frizzi, Riccardo Campi, and Sergio Serni

10.1   Introduction and History of Vaginal Mesh Implant

Surgical treatment of pelvic organ prolapse (POP) is very common in the female gender and is gradually increasing. Many women are living longer and have a high expectation for quality of life beyond menopause including an active lifestyle and the capacity for sexual activity.

POP can result either when defective genital support responds to normal intra-abdominal pressure or when normal pelvic organ supports are chronically exposed to high intra-abdominal pressures.

It is estimated that the lifetime risk of POP experiencing-related surgery ranges from 6.3 to 19% [1] and, among this group of women, 30% of them undergo one or more intervention for prolapse recurrence [2]. Some authors reported reoperation rates for recurrence after primary reconstructive surgery between 43 and 58% [3].

In an attempt to reduce the high incidence of surgical failures, to improve the quality of life of patients and to reconstruct the pelvic anatomy and rebalance the functionality of pelvic organs, until the early 1980s, gynaecologists began to implant prostheses for the stabilization of the pelvic floor. However, these prostheses were not specifically developed for POP treatment and were borrowed by those used for abdominal hernia's repair until the 1950s by general surgeons.

The principle that led the gynaecologists to use meshes for POP repair was inspired by general surgeons and allowed them to apply the same reconstructive principles of abdominal viscera's hernia repair.

The high success rate in abdominal hernia's surgery, the introduction in the mid-1990s of the first synthetic transvaginal sling for the correction of stress urinary incontinence (SUI) and later the popularity of the transobturator approach pushed the industry to produce specific materials for POP correction [4].

V. Li Marzi (✉) · J. Frizzi · R. Campi · S. Serni
Department of Urology, Careggi University Hospital, Florence, Italy

© Springer International Publishing AG, part of Springer Nature 2018   123
V. Li Marzi, M. Serati (eds.), *Management of Pelvic Organ Prolapse*,
Urodynamics, Neurourology and Pelvic Floor Dysfunctions,
https://doi.org/10.1007/978-3-319-59195-7_10

Indeed, in the first study in 1955 describing the use of meshes to repair cystocele, a tantalum mesh was used [5]. The researchers went on in identification of other materials suitable for use in humans, and in the 1970s the first report of xenogenous collagen mesh in urogynaecology was described [6]. In 1992, Zacharin described the use of excised vaginal epithelium (autologous tissue) as a free, full-thickness skin graft during surgery for recurrent POP [7].

In the 1980s and 1990s, first experiences with synthetic meshes were described from many authors, and several "homemade"-shaped meshes were placed with vaginal approach. An overview of the first studies describing the use of vaginal synthetic meshes for POP repair is shown in Table 10.1.

After the first attempts to use PTFE (Gore-Tex TM) meshes, the next step was the use of polypropylene mesh (Marlex®) derived from abdominal hernia's surgery. It was thereby used for the treatment of cystocele during the same period by several authors with good outcomes on POP repair [8–15], but controversial (or not reported) results regarding functional aspects and mesh-related complications [8–16].

As the interest from mesh manufacturers was increasingly growing, the first surgical mesh product specifically for use in POP was approved in 2002 by FDA (Food and Drug Administration) (Gynemesh PS TM Ethicon). Over the next few years, surgical mesh products for transvaginal POP repair became incorporated into "kits" that included tools to aid in the delivery and insertion of the mesh via the paravaginal space (Table 10.2).

Surgical mesh kits continued to evolve, adding new insertion tools, tissue fixation anchors, surgical techniques and absorbable and biologic materials. An increasing number of kits were introduced on the United States and European markets, pushed vigorously by industry, reaching in 2010 almost 100 devices on the

Table 10.1 Literature review of the first experiences with transvaginal synthetic prostheses for POP treatment

Authors/ year	N. pts	Mesh	Follow-up months	POP outcomes (%)	Mesh-related complications	References
Julian TM/1996	24	Polypropylene	24	100	25%	[8]
Flood CG/1998	142	Polypropylene	38	100	2.1%	[9]
Nicita G/1998	44	Polypropylene	13.9	93.2	0%	[10]
Mage P/1999	46	Polyester	26	100	2.1%	[11]
Migliari R/1999	15	Mixed fibre	23.4	93.4	–	[12]
Weber AM/2001	35	Polyglactin 910	23.3	42	–	[13]
Sand PK/2001	80	Polyglactin 910	12	75	–	[14]
Shah DK/2004	29	Polypropylene	25.1	94.1	0%	[15]

Table 10.2 Cornerstones in the urogynaecological synthetic prostheses employed for pelvic floor disorder treatment

Year		Pelvic floor disorders/ Company
1996	The FDA approved the first transvaginal mesh	SUI/Boston Scientific
1998	SUI surgery presents a revolutionary change with the introduction of tension-free vaginal tape (TVT)	SUI/Ethicon, Johnson & Johnson
2002	FDA approves the first surgical mesh for POP (Gynemesh PS™)	POP/Ethicon, Johnson & Johnson
2004	FDA approves the first transvaginal mesh kit (Apogee and Perigee)	POP/American Medical Systems (AMS)
2005	Ethicon started selling the Gynecare Prolift Kit in 2005 without marketing approval from the FDA. The FDA scolded J&J but approved the Prolift anyway in 2008	POP/Ethicon, Johnson & Johnson
2012	Ethicon announced that it would no longer manufacture and distribute vaginal mesh products (Prolift, Gynemesh) and minisling (TVT-Secur)	POP and SUI/Ethicon, Johnson & Johnson
2016	Endo International (Astora) suspended the production of vaginal mesh products (Elevate), medio-urethral sling (Monarc) and minisling (MiniArc)	POP and SUI/Endo International

market. The proposed advantages of kits are the reduced surgical trauma, the standardization of techniques, a faster learning curve and the use and ability to repair multiple compartments through a vaginal approach [17–20]. However, the initial studies, although underpowered and with a short follow-up, showed superior outcomes compared to traditional vaginal approaches in terms of POP recurrences [21].

These results were sufficient to let the meshes gain popularity among gynaecologists and urologists, who were not only motivated to improve outcomes in their patients but were also interested in adopting new surgical procedures in their existing, mostly narrow, surgical portfolio.

Given the high number of procedures performed for recurrences, it was not surprising that pelvic floor surgeons quickly placed vaginal mesh surgery within their therapeutic strategies for POP treatment [22].

Market data from manufacturers indicate that in 2010 approximately 300,000 women underwent surgical procedures in the United States to repair POP. According to industry estimates, approximately one out of three women receiving POP surgery underwent mesh placement, and three out of four (approximately 75,000) procedures were performed transvaginally.

This dramatic increase of mesh systems has led to a parallel increase of surgical complications. As such, in West Virginia there have been about 70,000 lawsuits for mesh's damages [23]. Moreover, the FDA has registered 3979 reports of injury and malfunction of the available surgical meshes between January 1, 2005 and December 31, 2010.

In 2008, FDA notified that adverse events after mesh placement were possible, albeit rare.

In 2011, following the finding that adverse events were increased, FDA made public the "safety warning", "Update on serious complications associated with transvaginal placement of surgical mesh for POP", identifying the use of vaginal mesh as a source of "continuing serious concern" [24–26].

In this update, FDA affirmed that the objective of the safety communication is to inform healthcare providers and patients that the risks of serious complications associated with transvaginal POP repair with mesh are not rare, contrary to what was stated in the 2008 Public Health Notification (PHN). This updated communication identified vaginal shortening, tightening and/or pain due to mesh contraction as a previously unidentified risk of transvaginal POP repair with mesh, and it provided recommendations for patients and healthcare providers [24]. Therefore, in 2011 FDA recommended cautious use of mesh for POP surgery as it was still unclear whether POP repair using synthetic meshes was or not superior to traditional vaginal surgery (Table 10.3).

The FDA statements initially generated great confusion in patients, physicians and media for several reasons. They did not mention that complications could occur also with traditional non-mesh repairs and therefore that their incidence might have been probably underestimated. Also, confusing mesh placement for POP repair with mesh placement for SUI led to a vicious cycle of misinformation from the media to the public opinion as, for example, most web information is lawsuit orientated rather than science orientated, with urogynaecologists and scientific associations running the risk of being relegated to a secondary role [27]. However, multiple factors may have contributed to this increase in complications, including increased use of urogynaecologic surgical mesh in the clinical community scenario, increased awareness on the potential adverse events associated with mesh repair after the 2008 PHN, an increased number of new POP meshes on the market or finally an increased number of actual adverse events associated with meshes [24].

Table 10.3 FDA warnings and communications about vaginal meshes

Year		
2008	FDA Health Notification	FDA publishes a communication to healthcare providers regarding complications associated with mesh used for POP and SUI
2011	FDA safety communication	FDA update of the safety communication is to inform healthcare providers and patients that the risks of serious complications associated with transvaginal POP repair with mesh are not rare, contrary to what was stated in the 2008 PHN
2012	FDA begins issuing 522 orders	FDA begins issuing 522 postmarket surveillance study orders to manufacturers of transvaginal mesh and minislings for POP and SUI
2016	Reclassification of surgical mesh for transvaginal POP repair	FDA is issuing a final order to reclassify surgical mesh for transvaginal POP repair from class II to class III
2017	522 postmarket surveillance study publications could begin	Publication of the first results of the 522 postmarket surveillance studies could begin in 2017

In 2015 even Scientific Committee on Emerging and Newly Identified Health Risks (SCENIHR) approved a document about "The safety of surgical meshes used in urogynecological surgery". The SCENIHR reported that clinical outcome following mesh implantation could be influenced by material properties, product design, overall mesh size, route of implantation, patient characteristics, associated procedures (e.g. hysterectomy) and the surgeon's experience. All these aspects should have then been taken into account when choosing the appropriate therapy [28].

In January 2016 FDA has issued its last "warning" about mesh surgery, in which the FDA's commission confirmed and strengthened what has already been reported in 2011. Surgical mesh for the transvaginal repair of POP has been definitively reclassified from class II to class III (high-risk devices) and required through a premarket approval application (PMA) the safety and efficacy of the mesh. These reclassifications by FDA are based on the determination that general controls and special controls together are not sufficient to provide reasonable assurance of safety and effectiveness. In addition, in the absence of an established positive benefit-risk profile, FDA has determined that the health's risk associated with the use of surgical mesh for transvaginal POP repair, also if previously identified, presents a potential unreasonable risk of illness or injury. Actually FDA does not believe there is sufficient evidence at this time to support the banning of this device. The safety and effectiveness of surgical mesh for transvaginal POP repair have not been established, and the collection of additional clinical evidence on these devices is needed. Such additional evidence may provide information to allow FDA to impose controls to mitigate the risks and more clearly characterize the benefits of these devices. In addition, FDA believes there are potential benefits from surgical mesh used for transvaginal POP repair including treatment of POP in appropriately selected women with severe or recurrent prolapse. FDA report concluded that the types of risks associated with transvaginal mesh for POP repair are similar across different vaginal compartments, and although mesh is an ideal anatomical support based on POP-Q stage, it is not a prerequisite for improvement in patient symptoms and in quality of life compared to native tissue repair.

FDA has modified the proposed identification for surgical mesh to clarify that the materials of construction may include synthetic material, non-synthetic material or their combination materials [29]. An important point to emphasize is that these warnings are expressed only about the transvaginal mesh and not for those implanted via transabdominal or for SUI treatment [27]. During these years many lawsuits have been filed against the producing companies with high economic losses and adverse publicity. As such, ligation against doctors and device companies has led many surgeons to stop using these devices. In June 2012, among mounting legal pressure and growing concern from the FDA, Ethicon announced that it would no longer manufacture and distribute vaginal mesh which sales made up a low percent of the company's revenue. Accordingly, in 2016 Endo International decided to stop selling Astora women's health products and close down the business. Surgeons, professional organizations and competitors were surprised by the decision undertaken by Endo International [22].

As a consequence, the surgical treatment of POP has been evolving, particularly in response to the FDA notifications about vaginal mesh and commercial decisions of interested companies [30]. Vaginal mesh procedures declined over time, comprising 27% of prolapse repairs in early 2008, 15% at the time of the first FDA notification regarding vaginal mesh, 5% by the second FDA notification and 2% at the end of 2011. The percentage of native tissue anterior/posterior repairs and apical suspensions increased, while the percentage of colpocleisis procedures remained constant [30]. There was a 25.5% increase in sacral colpopexy performed worldwide [31]. In an article published in 2015, 334 IUGA members responded to a survey. Most of the responses were from Europe (40%) and North America (23%). After the FDA safety communication regarding serious complications of using transvaginal mesh, 45% of responders reported decreased use of mesh, while 31% reported that it had no effect or that they did not use mesh for transvaginal prolapse (23.6%) [32]. Moreover, mesh revision surgery has increased over this same period. However, the exact underlying reasons for the changing surgical practice patterns are still unknown. Given the coincident timing between the FDA announcements and the pattern seen, it is possible that the FDA PHNs have been a major factor underlying this trend. Additionally, following the FDA PHN, the proliferation of legal activity directed at transvaginal mesh may also have had a significant impact on interest of both physicians and patients. Furthermore, though there was not an FDA-mandated recall of monofilament transvaginal mesh products, several manufacturers had voluntarily withdrawn their product from the marketplace, potentially reducing the mesh-related options available. Finally, an increased patient literacy regarding mesh and mesh-augmented repairs resulting from the widespread media attention and medicolegal activity may have had an effect on the number of individuals seeking revision of their implanted mesh, though this is purely speculative [33].

10.2 Why Should We Use Vaginal Mesh for POP Repair Today?

In 2016 a Cochrane review analysed 37 trials including 4023 women assessing the results of different correction techniques for POP of anterior segment [34]. Comparing permanent mesh versus native tissue repair, the prolapse's recurrence was significantly higher in conventional techniques compared to the use of polypropylene mesh implantation (RR 0.66, 95% CI 0.54–0.81, $I^2 = 3\%$). This suggests that if 19% of women are aware of POP after native tissue repair, between 10 and 15% will be aware of POP after permanent mesh repair. Rates of repeat surgery for POP were lower in the mesh group (RR 0.53, 95% CI 0.31–0.88, 12 RCTs, $I^2 = 0\%$). Moreover, recurrent POP on examination was less likely after mesh repair (RR 0.40, 95% CI 0.30–0.53, 21 RCTs, $I^2 = 73\%$). This suggests that if 38% of women have recurrent prolapse after native tissue repair, between 11 and 20% will do so after mesh repair.

In further two RCTs, the use of non-absorbable mesh vs. colporrhaphy in correcting anterior fascial defects showed best anatomical results with the use of mesh and no significant differences in outcomes (objective cure rate with mesh 12.9% vs. 39.6% for native tissue). Mesh procedures showed better prolapse symptom improvements than native tissue repairs (15% vs. 25.7%) [35, 36].

These results were also confirmed by more recent data published in the literature where women undergoing correction with synthetic mesh showed positive subjective and objective outcome with significant improvement in quality of life at a follow-up of 5 years [37].

Lamblin et al. have compared anterior colporrhaphy with vaginal colposuspension and transvaginal mesh (AMS Perigee transobturator anterior compartment repair system) in patients with symptomatic POP-Q stage 3 or 4 anterior vaginal wall prolapse. Although quality of life was improved overall in both groups, transobturator vaginal mesh gave better 2-year anatomical results than vaginal colposuspension. Mesh was particularly suitable for anterior vaginal wall repair [38].

Svabik et al. compared the efficacy of two standard surgical procedures, Prolift total vs. unilateral vaginal sacrospinous colpopexy with native tissue for posthysterectomy vaginal vault prolapse repair in patients with levator ani avulsion. They reported that sacrospinous fixation had a higher anatomical failure rate than the Prolift total repair after a 1-year follow-up [39].

Milani et al. compared the outcomes of synthetic mesh and native tissue surgery for the vaginal repair of POP. Anatomical and functional outcomes were reported as well as postoperative and de novo dyspareunia. For the anterior vaginal compartment, there was convincing evidence that the use of a synthetic mesh for the treatment of a prolapsed anterior vaginal wall was subjectively and objectively superior to a native tissue repair. There was, however, no difference in health-related quality of life between mesh and native tissue repair. The rate of de novo POP of the untreated vaginal compartment was significantly higher when synthetic mesh was used. There was also no evidence for a difference in the need for subsequent operations for POP or the occurrence of de novo dyspareunia or sexual function [40].

For the posterior vaginal compartment, there was moderate evidence that the use of mesh results in higher rates of objective cure and de novo POP of the anterior vaginal compartment, but no differences in subjective cure or de novo SUI [40].

For the treatment of more than one vaginal compartment, the meta-analysis showed that the use of mesh resulted in higher rates of subjective and objective "cure" but also in significantly higher rates of de novo POP of the untreated vaginal compartments. There were no differences in patient satisfaction, health-related quality of life, subsequent operations for POP, de novo dyspareunia, sexual function scores or de novo SUI. Mesh exposures, however, were frequently reported. The follow-ups of selected papers for that meta-analysis were mainly short (12 months) and sometimes medium-term (36 months) [40].

In the last Cochrane review is reported in case of anterior repair a mesh exposure rate of 10% (76/753), while mesh exposure in 17% (58/344) of the women after multi-compartment mesh repair [34].

Anyhow the problem of exposure/erosion should be seen in different views. More than one third (35%) of these exposures are minimal and asymptomatic, and they are often detected at a clinical control [24].

A further problem arises for posterior compartment defect repair. We have no currently robust studies which compared the results between traditional and median fascial plication of non-absorbable mesh implant. The few available trials indicate substantially no significant difference in short-term results between two methods [34].

However, a further aspect of debate arises when taking into consideration the anatomical studies of Fritsch et al. [41] about the nature of the rectovaginal fascia. This study highlighted that only dense connective tissue that is continuous with the adventitia with small rectal fat lobules interspersed between the slats. Therefore, it is unclear what surgeons are repairing with the fascial duplication. This aspect opens new research perspectives on the best treatment strategy for transvaginal correction of posterior compartment prolapse.

10.3   Why Should We *Not* Use Vaginal Mesh for POP Repair Today?

From 2008 to 2010, the most frequent complications reported by FDA about the use of surgical mesh devices included vaginal mesh erosion (also called exposure, extrusion or protrusion), shrinkage, pain (including painful sexual intercourse known as dyspareunia), infection, urinary problems (de novo SUI), bleeding and organ perforation (Fig. 10.1). There were also reports of recurrent prolapse, neuromuscular problems, vaginal scarring/shrinkage and emotional problems. Many of the medical device reporting cited the need for additional intervention, including medical or surgical treatment and hospitalization. Vaginal shrinkage was not reported in the previous 3-year period corresponding to the 2008 PHN.

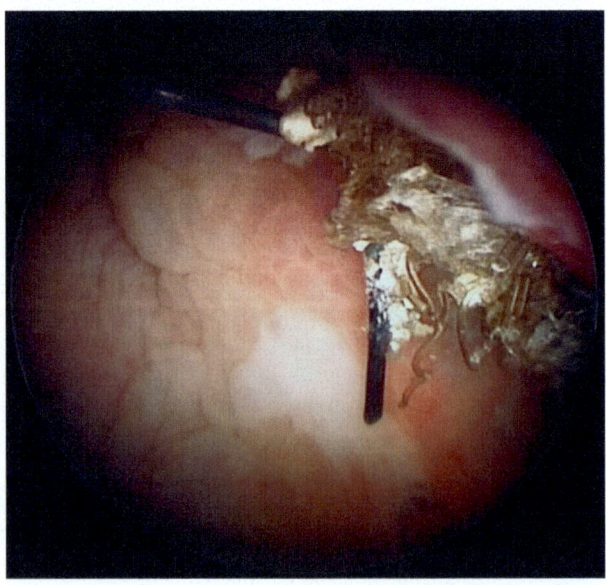

Fig. 10.1 Endoscopic view of erosion on the lateral bladder wall 4 years after vaginal mesh surgery

Between 2008 and 2010, there were seven reported deaths associated with POP repairs. Follow-up investigation on the death reports revealed that three of them were mesh-related (two bowel perforations, one haemorrhage). Four deaths were due to postoperative medical complications not directly related to the mesh placement procedure.

Meshes are associated with higher rates of repeat surgery SUI or mesh exposure and with higher rates of bladder injury at surgery and de novo SUI than native tissue repair. The risk-benefit profile means that transvaginal mesh has limited utility in primary surgery. While it is possible that in women with higher risk of recurrence, the benefits may outweigh the risks, there is currently no evidence to support this position [29].

A systematic review that included more than 7000 women concluded that abdominal POP surgery with mesh such as sacrocolpopexy resulted in lower rates of mesh complications compared to vaginal POP surgery with a median mesh erosion rate of 4% during a 2-year follow-up [42]. Vaginal surgery with mesh to correct apical prolapse is associated with a higher rate of complication requiring reoperation, when compared to sacrocolpopexy or traditional repair (7.2% vs. 4.8% vs. 1.9%, respectively) [43].

Anyway in this surgery the most important element to consider is not the anatomical result, but it is important to restore the function of the pelvic organs, restore the anatomy and also maintain a normal sexual function in sexually active women. In fact, it is an element that makes different the reconstruction of the abdominal wall by the reconstruction of the vaginal wall, and sexual function has absolutely to be taken into consideration [44]. The abdominal wall and its structures have less vascularization and innervation (scarcity of superficial and deep nervous receptors), appropriate to the function that it has to play.

The vaginal wall surface is constituted by a thin mucosa in which the epithelium, very sensitive to the sex hormones' blood levels, is rich in both arterial and venous vasculatures with an extremely high density of nervous receptors. It is therefore clear that surgery (employing synthetic mesh) may induce an important inflammatory reaction which can modify the healing and reconstruction of these tissues, creating an anomalous situation which sometimes weighs heavily on the women's sexual health and her physical and mental wellbeing [45].

10.4   When Should We Use Vaginal Mesh for POP?

Before proposing any surgery for POP repair, it must be taken into account that, on the one hand, the prolapse of pelvic organs represents an important condition that can severely affect the patient's quality of life but, on the other hand, it's a benign disease and therefore it never threats the woman's life. Any surgery should be therefore systematically addressed to solve problems, restoring normal function and anatomy leading to a significant improvement in quality of life, exposing the patient to the least possible risk of damages and complications. It is also known that a certain degree of prolapse (grades I–II) is physiological and almost always asymptomatic in women of a certain age [44].

As such, surgical treatment is indicated only in women with symptomatic POP and when conservative therapy proposals (pelvic floor rehabilitation, use of pessary, local hormone therapy) do not result in symptom improvement or are not accepted by the woman. Indications for the use of transvaginal mesh for POP reconstructive surgery are currently quite selected. Overall, transvaginal mesh placement is indicated in older, not sexually active patients, or as an alternative in specific cases of recurrence after primary standard vaginal surgery, or finally in patients where sacro-colpopexy is contraindicated.

The mesh implant should then be carefully evaluated, discussed and shared with the patient, individualizing the treatment in each case considering the disease's severity, the patient's age, the clinical history and the presence or not of factors that might potentially increase the risk of surgical complications (BMI > 30, diabetes, heavy smoking, vaginal atrophy, chronic steroid use, immunosuppressive therapy). Limiting factors are the young age constipation and chronic cough; those items will probably increase the risk of recurrence and therefore are to be evaluated, although they are not discriminating factor, especially in the case of mono-compartmental POP [37, 45]. Based on the above considerations, it is critical in current clinical practice to counsel properly women with POP explaining the success rates reported in the literature, the available surgical techniques and the surgeon's success rate. Moreover, the mesh-related complications should be explained carefully.

Another element to consider is the possible reaction of hypersensitivity to synthetic mesh. This reaction, shown by the presence of humoral markers of lymphocyte activation, was detected in one case-control study and a limited number of women, but the increase in allergic reactions in the general population may reasonably increase these events. Then, even if not predictable, implantation of the mesh should be used with caution in patients with severe allergic diathesis or autoimmune diseases [46].

A relevant aspect to consider in this type of surgery is the role of surgeon experience. Indeed, many studies showed a strong correlation between reduced surgeon's experience and greater frequency of complications (2.9 vs. 15.6%) [47, 48]. The surgical capacity plays a decisive role in lower incidence of complications; accordingly, this type of surgery should be performed in specialized centres with high surgical volume and only by trained pelvic surgeons [45, 47]. Recurrent errors in surgical technique are most common in low-experienced surgeon, increasing the mesh's erosion risks. Among these, the most frequent are exposure, mesh surface positioning (without the so-called full-thickness dissection), the trimming of the incision edges in the vaginal wall (who must maintain a certain laxity) and excessive tension of the mesh, especially if concomitant hysterectomy is performed with "T" incision of the vaginal wall.

Liang et al. evaluated the impact of mesh implantation on vaginal collagen and elastin metabolism in nonhuman primates. In an attempt to ascertain whether differences in erosion rates were caused by mesh positions, which was transvaginally or abdominally placed [49], Noblett et al. found that abdominal sacrocolpopexy and full-thickness vaginal dissection resulted in histologically similar locations and that using a full-thickness dissection technique for transvaginal mesh might be one way of reducing mesh exposure rates [50].

10.5   When Should We Use Vaginal Biological Graft for POP Repair?

As an alternative to synthetic prostheses, biological grafts have been proposed in recent years as they may have a lower risk of erosion or infection. However, evidence on efficacy is insufficient mainly on long-term [34].

Cadaveric fascia lata with or without pubovaginal sling has been utilized to correct anterior compartment POP with a success rate varying from 81 to 100% with satisfactory complication rates [51].

Leboeuf et al. reviewed 24 women with native tissue POP repair and 19 with porcine dermis POP repair. At 15-month follow-up, the success rate was 100% and 84% in the first group and in the group with porcine dermis graft, respectively [52].

Meschia et al. in a multicentre randomized clinical trial compared the anterior colporrhaphy and anterior colporrhaphy augmented with porcine dermis. The success rate at 1 year was 93% in the anterior colporrhaphy with porcine graft intersection group as compared to 81% in anterior colporrhaphy group with a 1% rate of graft erosion [53].

In one another RCT, Natale et al. compared polypropylene mesh with porcine dermis. At 2 years, significantly fewer women had anterior vaginal wall recurrence in the mesh group compared to the porcine graft group (28% vs. 44%). Mesh erosion was reported in 6.3% following surgery. The authors reported superior sexual activity results in the porcine graft group as compared to polypropylene mesh group ($p = 0.03$) [54].

Feldner et al. compared anterior colporrhaphy with small intestine submucosa (SIS) graft in a RCT and reported an objective failure rate of 33% after anterior colporrhaphy that was significantly higher in comparison with 14% in the SIS group [55].

Moreover, Menefee et al. in a RCT compared three surgical procedures, anterior colporrhaphy, vaginal paravaginal repair using porcine dermis graft and vaginal paravaginal with "homemade"-shaped polypropylene mesh, and also reported a higher objective success rate after the polypropylene mesh as compared to the porcine dermis group (86% vs. 52%) and to the anterior colporrhaphy group (86% vs. 53%). The subjective failure rate was not significantly different and was 3.4, 12 and 13%, respectively. The graft erosion rate was 4.3% in the porcine dermis group and 13.8% in the mesh group [56].

In a recent Cochrane review on the surgical management of anterior compartment prolapse, eight trials compared anterior colporrhaphy with several biological grafts (porcine dermis, small intestine submucosa, cadaveric fascia lata, bovine pericardium). There were no differences detected between porcine dermis graft or small intestine submucosa and anterior colporrhaphy for the primary outcomes of awareness of POP, POP on examination and reoperation for POP. Biological grafts had similar outcomes to anterior colporrhaphy in awareness of POP and reoperation for prolapse; however, the recurrent anterior POP rate on examination was less after biological graft repair as compared to anterior colporrhaphy (RR 0.74, 95% CI 0.55–0.99 $n = 646$, $I^2 = 29\%$, low-quality evidence) [34].

10.6 Concluding Remarks

The aims of reconstructive pelvic surgery are to restore anatomy, to maintain or restore normal bowel and bladder function and to maintain vaginal capacity for sexual intercourse. It is then crucial to know the patient's goals prior to surgery in order to have an optimal outcome.

When planning a surgical procedure to treat POP, addressing the vaginal apex is key, as many reports validated the role that apical support plays in overall normal pelvic anatomy and successful surgical outcomes.

Screening and testing patients for other pelvic floor disorders (urinary incontinence, voiding dysfunction, faecal incontinence, difficulty defecating) are critical prior to surgical treatment. Uterine-sparing procedures are becoming more popular, and encouraging data are supporting their role in reconstructive pelvic surgery [57–59].

However, there is no ideal surgical technique for the treatment of POP, and, to date, the ideal mesh, able to restrict the anatomy and functionality of the pelvic organs with no or minimal potential risks for the woman, does still not exist.

In this scenario, the exact role of meshes remains controversial even though many patients continue to benefit from them. As mesh-related complications constitute the major drawback to their use, preventing them will be the greatest challenge in coming years. Healing failures requires an in-depth assessment, with recognition of the role and importance of host factors that are detrimental to healing. Surgical techniques, training, proper patient selection and materials still need to be improved [27]. It is also of utmost importance an appropriate patient selection and counselling in order to achieve optimal outcomes of all surgical procedures.

Overall, to date, the implantation of any mesh for the treatment of POP via the vaginal route should be only considered in complex cases in particular after failed primary repair surgery or expected fail surgery [28].

Future research will lead to identify materials and techniques that increasingly approach the concept of "ideal" prosthesis for POP repair. Moreover, a key step forward to improve outcomes of transvaginal POP repair will be to overcome the concept of vaginal mesh placement as "easy and fast" that was claimed by industries and manufacturers in the past. Indeed, FDA has never expressed specific contraindications to the use of mesh, but instead it has highlighted recommendations for their proper use. To standardize techniques, to improve patient outcomes avoiding mesh-related complications and to treat such complications in the best way, a key step will be to concentrate this type of surgery in specialized high-volume centres with great experience in POP surgery that can translate the knowledge to the future generations of pelvic surgeons. As such, some authors even recommend the introduction of specific certification systems for specialists and "fellow" trainees based on existing international guidelines and established in cooperation with the relevant international surgical associations [28]. An interesting survey of AUA's (American Urological Association) members showed that 31.9% of surveyed urologists reported that they had not received any formal training in mesh placement (in forms of either fellowship or at residency level), and only two-thirds of urologists that attended industry-sponsored courses received any type of hands-on training (including cadaver or simulator training) [60]. Keys et al. described the hazard of reoperation for complications was only lower for patients treated by very high-volume surgeons [60]. In accordance with these concepts, more recently, a consensus statement of the European Association of Urology and the European Urogynaecological Association has been published in which the mesh use is recommended for POP only in complex cases and limited to those surgeons with appropriate training [61]. Moreover, women should be adequately informed regarding the reported success rates and the potential mesh-related adverse events compared with non-mesh alternatives, at both a literature and surgeon level, and should therefore be actively involved in the decision-making process [61].

The possibility to use stem cells for the regeneration of tissues (TERM—tissue-engineered repair material), as is already done experimentally for the treatment of SUI to regenerate the urethral sphincter, represents a potential future perspective in the repair of the damaged native tissue and may provide new alternatives to native tissue repair or mesh repair for POP [62].

Current use of mesh in transvaginal POP surgery is perfectible, and in order to reduce potential adverse effects and complications, research for the ideal mesh material is ongoing. However, it is critical to highlight that surgeons and institutions treating POP should offer both transvaginal and transabdominal (especially minimally invasive) approaches in order to offer patients a personalized approach that is tailored to the POP's and patient's characteristics.

References

1. Olsen AL, Smith VJ, Bergstrom JO, et al. Epidemiology of surgical managed pelvic organ prolapse and urinary incontinence. Obstet Gynecol. 1997;89:501.
2. Porges RF, Smilen SW. Long term analysis of the surgical management of pelvic support defects. Am J Obstet Gynecol. 1994;171(6):1518–26.
3. Smith FJ, Holman CD, Moorin RE, et al. Lifetime risk of undergoing surgery for pelvic organ prolapse. Obstet Gynecol. 2010;116:1096.
4. Witheside JL, Weber AM, Meyn LA, et al. Risk fctors for prolapse recurrence after vaginal repair. Am J Obstet Gyncol. 2004;191:1533–8.
5. Moore J, Armstrong JT, Willis SH. The use of tantalum mesh in cystocele with critical report of ten cases. Am J Obstet Gynecol. 1955;69(5):1127–35.
6. Friedman EA, Meltzer RM. Collagen mesh prosthesis for repair of endopelvic fascial defects. Am J Obstet Gynecol. 1970;106(3):430–3.
7. Zacharin RF. Free full-thickness vaginal epithelium graft in correction of recurrent genital prolapse. Aust N Z J Obstet Gynaecol. 1992;32(2):146–8.
8. Julian TM. The efficacy of Marlex mesh in the repair of severe, recurrent vaginal prolapse of the anterior midvaginal wall. Am J Obstet Gynecol. 1996;175(6):1472–5.
9. Flood CG, Drutz HP, Waja L. Anterior colporrhaphy reinforced with Marlex mesh for the treatment of cystoceles. Int Urogynecol J Pelvic Floor Dysfunct. 1998;9(4):200–4.
10. Nicita G. A new operation for genitourinary prolapse. J Urol. 1998;160(3 Pt 1):741–5.
11. Mage P. Interposition of a synthetic mesh by vaginal approach in the cure of genital prolapse. J Gynecol Obstet Biol Reprod. 1999;28(8):825–9.
12. Migliari R, Usai E. Treatment results using a mixed fiber mesh in patients with grade IV cystocele. J Urol. 1999;161(4):1255–8.

13. Weber AM, Walters MD, Piedmonte MR, Ballard LA. Anterior colporrhaphy: a randomized trial of three surgical techniques. Am J Obstet Gynecol. 2001;185(6):1299–304; discussion 1304-6.
14. Sand PK, Koduri S, Lobel RW, Winkler HA, Tomezsko J, Culligan PJ, Goldberg R. Prospective randomized trial of polyglactin 910 mesh to prevent recurrence of cystoceles and rectoceles. Am J Obstet Gynecol. 2001;184(7):1357–62; discussion 1362-4.
15. Shah DK, Paul EM, Rastinehad AR, Eisenberg ER, Badlani GH. Short-term outcome analysis of total pelvic reconstruction with mesh: the vaginal approach. J Urol. 2004;171(1):261–3.
16. Lensen EJM, et al. Surgical treatment of pelvic organ prolapse: a historical review with emphasis on the anterior compartment. Int Urogynecol J. 2013;24:1593–602.
17. Committee on Gynecologic Practice. Committee Opinion no.513: vaginal placement of synthetic mesh for pelvic organ prolapse. Ostet Gynecol. 2011;118(6):1459–64.
18. Chen CC, Ridgeway B, Paraiso MF. Biologic grafts and synthetic meshes in pelvic reconstructive surgery. Clin Obstet Gynecol. 2007;50(2):383–411.
19. Amid PK. Classification of biomaterials and their related complications in abdominal wall hernia surgery. Hernia. 1997;1:15–21.
20. Rogo-Gupta L, Rodriguez LV, Litwin MS, et al. Trends in surgical mesh use for pelvic organ prolapse from 2000 to 2010. Ostet Gynecol. 2012;120(5):1105–15.
21. Sliva WA, Karram MM. Scientific basis for use of grafts during vaginal reconstructive procedures. Curr Opin Obstet Gynecol. 2005;17(5):519–29.
22. Roovers J-P. Collaboration with the mesh industry: who needs who. Int Urogynecol J. 2016;27:1293–5. https://doi.org/10.1007/s00192-016-3075-8.
23. Jonsson Funk M, Edenfield AL, Pate V, et al. Trends in use of surgical mesh for pelvic organ prolapse. Am J Obstet Gynecol. 2013;208(1):79–97.
24. FDA safety communication. UPDATE on serious complications associated with transvaginal placement of surgical mesh for pelvic organ prolapse. Silver Spring; FDA July 27, 2011.
25. FDA Executive Summary Surgical mesh for the treatment of women with pelvic organ prolapse and stress incontinence; Obstetric and Gynecology Devices Advisory Committee Meeting; 2011. Sept 8.
26. ACOG. Joint recommendations issued on use of vaginal mesh for POP. November 21, 2011.
27. Costantini E, Lazzeri M. What part does mesh play in urogenital prolapse management? Curr Opin Urol. 2015;25:300–4.
28. SCENIHR Opinion on The safety of surgical meshes used in urogynecologicalsurgery. The SCENIHR approved this Opinion on 3 December 2015.
29. FDA Strengthens requirement for surgical mesh for the tranvaginal repair of POP to address safety risks- Janury 4, 2016.
30. Skoczylas LC, Turner LC, Wang L, Winger DG, Shepherd JP. Changes in prolapse surgery trends relative to FDA notifications regarding vaginal mesh. Int Urogynecol J. 2014;25(4):471–7. https://doi.org/10.1007/s00192-013-2231-7.
31. Haya N, Baessler K, Christmann-Schmid C, et al. Prolapse and continence surgery in countries of the organization for economic cooperation and development in 2012. Am J Obstet Gynecol. 2015;212:755.
32. Ghoniem G, Hammett J. Female pelvic medicine and reconstructive surgery practice patterns: IUGA member survey. Int Urogynecol J. 2015;26(10):1489–94. https://doi.org/10.1007/s00192-015-2734-5. Epub 2015 May 28
33. Younger A, Rac G, Clemens JQ, Kobashi K, Nitti V, Jacobs I, Lemack GE, Brown ET, Dmochowski R, Maclachlan L. Pelvic organ prolapse surgery in academic female pelvic medicine and reconstructive surgery urology practice in the setting of the food and drug administration public health notifications. Urology. 2016;91:46–51. https://doi.org/10.1016/j.urology.2015.12.057.
34. Maher C, Feiner B, Baessler K, et al. Transvaginal mesh or grafts compared with native tissue repair for vaginal prolapse (Review). Cochrane Database Syst Rev. 2016;11:CD004014.
35. Nieminen K, Hiltunen R, Takala T, et al. Outcomes after anterior vaginal wall repair with mesh: a randomized controlled trial with 3 year follow-up. Am J Obstet Gynecol. 2010;203(3):235–8.

36. Rudnicki M, Laurikainen E, Pogosean R, et al. A 3-year follow-up after anterior colporraphy compared with collagen coated transvaginal mesh for anterior vaginal wall prolapse: a randomised controlled trial. BJOG. 2016;123(1):136–42.
37. Meyer I, McGwin G, Swain TA, et al. Synthetic graft augmentation in vaginal prolapse surgery: long-term objective and subjective outcomes. J Minim Invasive Gynecol. 2016;23:616–21.
38. Lamblin G, Van-Nieuwenhuyse A, Chabert P, et al. A randomized controlled trial comparing anatomical and functional outcome between vaginal colposuspension and transvaginal mesh. Int Urogynecol J. 2014;25:961–70.
39. Svabik K, Martan A, Masata J, et al. Comparison of vaginal mesh repair with sacrospinous vaginal colpopexy in the management of vaginal vault prolapse after hysterectomy in patients with levator ani avulsion: a randomized controlled trial. Ultrasound Obstet Gynecol. 2014;43:365–71.
40. Milani AL, Vollebregt A, Roovers JP, Withagen MIJ. The use of mesh in vaginal prolapse. Ned Tijdschr Geneeskd. 2013;157(31):A6324. Review.
41. Fritsch H, Lienemann A, Brenner E, et al. Clinical anatomy of the pelvic floor. Adv Anat Embryol Cell Biol. 2004;175:III–X, 1-64.
42. Jia X, Glazener C, Mowatt G, Jenkinson D, Fraser C, Bain C, Burr J. Systematic review of the efficacy and safety of using mesh in surgery for uterine or vaginal vault prolapse. Int Urogynecol J. 2010;21(11):1413–31.
43. Diwadkar GB, Barber MD, Feiner B, Maher C, Jelovsek JE. Complication and reoperation rates after apical vaginal prolapse surgical repair: a systematic review. Obstet Gynecol. 2009;113(2 Pt 1):367–73.
44. Ellington DR, Richter HE. Indications, Controindications, and Complications of mesh in surgical Treatment of Peelvic Organ Prolapse. Clin Obstet Gynecol. 2013;56(2):276–88.
45. Dallenbach P. To mesh or not to mesh: a review of pelvic organ reconstruttive surgery. Int J Womens Health. 2015;7:331–43.
46. Wang AC, Lee L, Lin CT, et al. A istologic and immunohistochemical analysis of defective vaginal healing after continence taping procedures: a prospective case-controlled pilot study. Am J Obstet Gynecol. 2004;191:1868–74.
47. Barski D, Otto T, Gerullis H. Systematic review and classification of complications after anterior, posterior, apical and total vaginal mesh implantation for prolapse repair. Surg Technol Int. 2014;24:217–24.
48. Achtari C, Hiscock R, O'Reilly BA, et al. Risk factors for mesh erosion after transvaginal surgery using polypropilene or composite polypropilene mesh. Int Uroynecol J Pelvic Floor Dyfunct. 2005;16(5):389–94.
49. Liang R, Zong W, Palcsey S, et al. Impact of prolapse meshes on the metabolism of vaginal extracellular matrix in rhesus macaque. Am J Obstet Gynecol. 2015;212:174.e1–e17.
50. Noblett K, Brueseke T, Lin F, Rosenblatt P. Comparison of location of mesh placed transvaginally vs mesh placed abdominally at the time of sacrocolpopexy. Int Urogynecol J. 2015;26:79–83.
51. Maher C, et al. Pelvic organ prolapse surgery. In: Abrams P, Cardozo L, Wagg A, Wein A, editors. Incontinence: 6th International Consultation on Incontinence. Tokyo 2016; 2017. p. 1855–991.
52. Leboeuf L, Miles RA, Kim SS, Gousse AE. Grade 4 cystocele repair using 4-defect repair and porcine xenograft acellular matrix (Pelvicol). Outcome measures using SEAPI. Urology. 2004;64(2):282–6.
53. Meschia M, Pifarotti P, Bernasconi F, et al. Porcine skin collagen implants to prevent anterior vaginal wall prolapse recurrence: a multicenter, randomized study. J Urol. 2007;177(1):192–5.
54. Natale F, La Penna C, Padoa A, et al. A prospective, randomized, controlled study comparing Gynemesh, a synthetic mesh, and Pelvicol, a biologic graft, in the surgical treatment of recurrent cystocele. Int Urogynecol J Pelvic Floor Dysfunct. 2009;20(1):75–81.
55. Feldner PC, Castro RA, Cipolotti LA, et al. Anterior vaginal wall prolapse: a randomized controlled trial of SIS graft versus traditional colporrhaphy. Int Urogynecol J Pelvic Floor Dysfunct. 2010;21(9):1057–63.

56. Menefee SA, Dyer KY, Lukacz ES, et al. Colporrhaphy compared with mesh or graft-reinforced vaginal paravaginal repair for anterior vaginal wall prolapse: a randomized controlled trial. Obstet Gynecol. 2011;118:1337–44.
57. Maldonado PA, Wai CY. Pelvic organ prolapse new concepts in pelvic floor anatomy. Obstet Gynecol Clin North Am. 2016;43(1):15–26.
58. Lee U, Raz S. Emerging concepts for pelvic organ prolapse surgery: what is cure? Curr Urol Rep. 2011;12(1):62–7.
59. Elliott CS, Yeh J, Comiter CV, Chen B, Sokol ER. The predictive value of a cystocele for concomitant vaginal apical prolapse. J Urol. 2013;189(1):200–3.
60. Keys T, Campeau L, Badlani G. Synthetic mesh in the surgical repair of pelvic organ prolapse: current status and future directions. Urology. 2012;80:237–43.
61. Chapple CR, Cruz F, Deffieux X, et al. Consensus statement of the European Urology Association and the European Urogynaecological Association on the use of implanted materials for treating pelvic organ prolapse and stress urinary incontinence. Eur Urol. 2017;72(3):424–31. https://doi.org/10.1016/j.eururo.2017.03.048.
62. Boennelycke M, Gras S, Lose G. Tissue engineering as a potential alternative or adjunct to surgical reconstruction in treating pelvic prolapse. Int Urogynecol J. 2013;24(5):741–7.

Posterior Prolapse Repair: The Evolution of the Surgical Approach

Marco Soligo

In the light of the historical perspective described by Cundiff et al. (1998), the long lasting tradition on posterior repair can be appreciated [1]. It was the early nineteenth century when the first report became apparent: Fricke JC in 1833 described *elytrorrhaphy* as a technique to denudate and close the posterior vaginal wall to repair genital prolapse. Then Simon G. in 1867 firstly introduced the term *posterior colporrhaphy* as a more aggressive levator ani muscle plication in the inferior vaginal portion to create an inferior shelf and a superior pocket. The same concept was then adopted by Hegar (1870) who introduced the *colpoperineorrhaphy* with the classic triangular denudation of the perineal body.

In the nineteenth century, the actual target of posterior repair was generically the genital prolapse. In the absence of clear anatomical and physiopathogenetic understanding, *colpoperineorrhaphy* was not only adopted for posterior vaginal defects, but it was considered as the unique solution to the genital prolapse; in fact the surgical goals of *colpoperineorrhaphy* are constriction of the vaginal tube, creation of a perineal shelf, and partially closing the genital hiatus.

Looking at posterior repair in an historical perspective, one can recognize a subtle redline of ignorance and misconception characterizing the surgical approach in different eras. The **first point of this redline** is the fact that for a long period of time, colpoperineorrhaphy was addressed to the treatment of all forms of genital prolapse.

Later on, a better anatomical understanding prompted the distinction of the genital prolapse into different vaginal segments, i.e., anterior, central, and posterior, leading to the development of different surgical techniques for every different compartment.

M. Soligo
Urogynecology Unit, Obstetrics and Gynecology Department, Buzzi Hospital ASST-FBF-Sacco Milan, University of Milan, Milan, Italy
e-mail: marcosoligo@fastwebnet.it

© Springer International Publishing AG, part of Springer Nature 2018
V. Li Marzi, M. Serati (eds.), *Management of Pelvic Organ Prolapse*,
Urodynamics, Neurourology and Pelvic Floor Dysfunctions,
https://doi.org/10.1007/978-3-319-59195-7_11

Despite this, the traditional approach to the posterior repair has little changed through decades, with the major difference consisting in avoiding the muscular involvement in the most cranial aspects of tissue duplication to reduce postoperative pain and dyspareunia. In the twentieth century, the problem of a correct definition of the bulging of the posterior vaginal wall was not felt as such by gynecologists, which generically termed this condition as "rectocele." This term become so popular that it resisted through years and criticism [2] remaining so far the most adopted term to recall the posterior vaginal wall relaxation and correlates [3].

In the beginning of the second half of the last century, some authors started to claim a high level of dyspareunia after traditional posterior colporrhaphy, and it was until 1978 when Kahn and Stanton added the observation of a higher level of defecatory disorders.

This awareness was perfectly in line with contemporary developing concepts of the medical approach to diseases, raising attention to the patient as a whole. In 1948 the World Health Organization (WHO) introduced in its constitution a broader definition of health as "a state of complete physical, mental, and social well-being and not merely the absence of disease or infirmity" [4, 2]. Also David L. Sackett et al. in his famous letter to BMJ in 1996 titled *Evidence based medicine: what it is and what it isn't* quote philosophical origins of evidence-based medicine, back to midnineteenth century and earlier [5].

In this context has to be placed the beginning of a more comprehensive approach to the anatomical and functional disorders of the posterior vaginal compartment (incidentally the anterior rectal compartment for colorectal surgeons). In fact Redding in 1961, as the first among colorectal surgeons, suggested to add a posterior repair while surgically dealing with other anorectal disorders, and Marks in 1967 comes out in *Diseases of the Colon and Rectum* with a paper titling *The rectal side of the rectocele* [6, 7]. He appropriately pointed out the high rate of defecatory complaints after posterior vaginal repair and claimed a concomitant *transanal approach* to reduce redundant rectal mucosa. Since then, many authors advocated a *transanal approach* to the so-called rectocele, claiming a success rate of up to 85% [8–11].

Here, once again, **our redline** comes out: from colorectal literature it is implied that surgeon's endpoint was merely functional, having the improvement of defecatory disorders as an outcome. On the other side, gynecologists were focusing exclusively on anatomical vaginal restoration. This incredible misunderstanding persisted for a long period of time generating considerable confusion. A direct comparison between different approaches was then necessary. As clearly pointed out by Karram and Maher (2013) in their recent review on *Surgery for posterior vaginal wall prolapse*, the *vaginal approach* resulted superior to *transanal* repair of rectocele in terms of anatomical restoration of the vagina, and in some cases also in functional terms [3].

As a matter of fact, the vaginal approach to posterior defects gained good results, being effective in anatomical restoration in a range between 76 and 96% with a dyspareunia rate of 18% and difficult defecation of 26% [3].

Between the years 1980 and 1990 of the past century, the traditional posterior repair had been challenged by the concept of a *site-specific defect repair*, claiming that every single fascial defect should be surgically addressed. Once more, a direct comparison between techniques highlighted the superiority of midline fascial plication over the discrete approach [12, 13].

Coming into the new century, the concept of functional disorders (i.e., sexual or defecatory) associated with pelvic organ prolapse (POP) becomes increasingly accepted also in the case of a posterior vaginal wall descent. Colpocystodefecography, functional magnetic resonance, and more recently ultrasound imaging added a morphological background to this concept showing a wide range of possible morphological bowel abnormalities in association with defecatory disorders. At the same time, some authors raised the attention to the fact that abnormal morphological findings are quite common in asymptomatic subjects [14]. We will come back to these aspects in a while.

Commenting on surgical approaches to the posterior repair, what came with the spring out of the new millennium has to be cited: the new era of *transvaginal mesh*, as a possible solution to deficient tissue consistency in women with genital prolapse. The rationale behind this strategy was a supposed excessive failure rate of traditional fascial reconstructive surgery: the worst results in surgical series were adopted to claim for the new approach. Therefore transvaginal meshes had been adopted also to correct the posterior compartment of the pelvic floor. The 2008 NICE report over nine studies (3 RCTs, 417 patients) observed a statistically nonsignificant difference in anatomical failure rate between augmented and non-augmented posterior repair (20% vs. 14%, respectively) with a 14% rate of mesh erosion [15]. More recently the Cochrane Systematic Review by Maher et al. (2016) states that "The risk-benefit profile means that transvaginal mesh has limited utility in primary surgery [16]. While it is possible that in women with higher risk of recurrence the benefits may outweigh the risks, there is currently no evidence to support this position." At present, little room remain for transvaginal mesh adoption, until substantial innovation will come from materials technology.

As an alternative, an *abdominal approach* (laparoscopic or robotic) can be considered with a success rate ranging between 45 and 91% [3]. The interest of this approach is mainly in the possibility of addressing composite surgical targets including defecatory dysfunction, after mandatory in-depth colorectal investigation [17].

In the first decade of the new century, more and more gynecologist introduced in their current clinical POP assessment a bowel history taken and in case of dysfunction colpocystodefecography, anorectal manometry and/or endoanal ultrasound. A multidisciplinary approach has become more popular, with colorectal surgeons increasingly involved in clinical assessment of women with multi-compartment disorders leading to different timing for surgeries, transanal vs. transvaginal first or vice versa, or, in some instances, to a combination surgery (transanal and transvaginal) approach.

The **redline** comes out again when awareness of concomitant functional disorders prompted gynecologists and colorectal surgeons to overemphasize the role of anatomical defects as responsible for the disorders they were examining. Unfortunately, the complexity of possible combinations between different anatomical findings (rectoceles, enteroceles, sigmoidoceles, rectal intussusception, rectal-anal intussusception, rectal prolapse, and solitary rectal ulcer syndrome) with different functional disorders (slow transit constipation or defecatory disorders, including dyssynergic defecation) makes the clinical approach to these disorders a complex one. *Consistently Inconsistent, the Posterior Vaginal Wall* is the eloquent title of a recent (2016) publication from Hale and Fenner. A careful reading of that paper is warmly recommended to those wishing to deal with posterior pelvic floor disorders. It is fully evident that every single case has to be thoroughly investigated and addressed conservatively first. Surgery remains the last step in the treatment algorithm [17].

In conclusion the paper from Hale and Fenner (2016) also introduces a key concept for the future: the patient.

It becomes more and more evident that the outcome of surgery can't be simply anatomical and/or functional. The impact of the disease on health-related quality of life (HRQoL), patient's expectations from surgery, and patient-reported outcomes (PRO) should all be added to objective anatomical and functional data to determine a "composite outcome" measurement [18].

References

1. Cundiff GW, Weidner AC, Visco AC, et al. An anatomic and functional assessment of the discrete defect rectocele repair. Am J Obstet Gynecol. 1998;179(6 pt 1):1451–6.
2. Soligo M. Posterior pelvic floor dysfunction: there is an immediate need to standardize terminology. Int Urogynecol J Pelvic Floor Dysfunct. 2007;18(4):369–71.
3. Karram M, Maher C. Surgery for posterior vaginal wall prolapse. Int Urogynecol J. 2013;24:1835–41.
4. World Health Organization. *WHO definition of Health*, Preamble to the Constitution of the World Health Organization as adopted by the International Health Conference, New York, 19–22 June 1946; signed on 22 July 1946 by the representatives of 61 States (Official Records of the World Health Organization, no. 2, p. 100) and entered into force on 7 April 1948. In: Grad FP (2002), "The Preamble of the Constitution of the World Health Organization". Bull World Health Organ. 80(12): 982.
5. Sackett DL, Rosenberg WM, Gray JA, et al. Evidence based medicine: what it is and what it isn't. BMJ. 1996;312:71–2.
6. Redding MD. The relaxed perineum and anorectal disease. Dis Colon Rectum. 1965;8:279–81.
7. Marks MM. The rectal side of the rectocele. Dis Colon Rectum. 1967;10:387–8.
8. Sullivan ES, Leaverton GH, Hardwick CE. Transrectal perineal repair: an adjunct to improved function after anorectal surgery. Dis Colon Rectum. 1968;11:196–14.
9. Sehapayak S. Transrectal repair of rectocele: an extended armamentarium of colorectal surgeons: a report of 355 cases. Dis Colon Rectum. 1985;28:422–33.
10. Khubchandani IT, Clancy JP III, Rosen L, Riether RD, Stasik JJJ. Endorectal repair of rectocele revisited. Br J Surg. 1997;84(1):89–91.
11. Arnold MW, Stewart WR, Aguilar PS. Rectocele repair four years' experience. Dis Colon Rectum. 1990;33(8):684–7.
12. Abramov Y, Gandhi S, Goldberg RP, Botros SM, Kwon C, Sand PK. Site-specific rectocele repair compared with standard posterior colporrhaphy. Obstet Gynecol. 2005;105(2):314–8.
13. Paraiso MF, Jelovsek JE, Frick A, Chen CC, Barber MD. Laparoscopic compared with robotic sacrocolpopexy for vaginal prolapse: a randomized controlled trial. Obstet Gynecol. 2011;118(5):1005–13.

14. Palit S, Bhan C, Lunniss PJ, et al. Evacuation proctography: a reappraisal of normal variability. Colorectal Dis. 2014;16(7):538–46.
15. National Institute for Health and Care Excellence (NICE). Surgical repair of vaginal wall prolapse using mesh. London: NICE; 2008.
16. Maher C, Feiner B, Baessler K, et al. Transvaginal mesh or grafts compared with native tissue repair for vaginal prolapse (Review). Cochrane Database Syst Rev. 2016;(2):CD012079. https://doi.org/10.1002/14651858.CD012079.
17. Hale DS, Fenner D. Consistently inconsistent, the posterior vaginal wall. Am J Obstet Gynecol. 2016;214(3):314–20.
18. Srikrishna S, Robinson D, Cardozo L, Thiagamoorthy G. Patient and surgeon goal achievement 10 years following surgery for pelvic organ prolapse and urinary incontinence. Int Urogynecol J. 2015;26:1679–86.

The Role of Hysterectomy in Genitourinary Prolapse

Maurizio Serati and Paola Sorice

Currently the role of hysterectomy in the surgical strategy of POP repair remains controversial. This is a topic of discussion in the scientific world, and many studies that would like to make light on the situation are coming out in the next years.

The last version of the ICI report included a comment on the role of hysterectomy in the surgical repair of pelvic organ prolapse (POP) "…hysterectomy at the time of POP repair is the standard practice in most parts of the world despite the fact that descent of the uterus may be a consequence, not a cause of POP. Surprisingly, given its widespread use, concomitant hysterectomy is not an evidence-based practice." [1]. This last statement emphatically paraphrases one of the strongest debates on the topic of POP surgery. In 1934, Bonney first suggested that the "Uterus has passive role in uterovaginal prolapse." Many years later, in 1996, Nichols concluded that "A dropped uterus is the result and not the cause of a genital prolapse" [2]. However, in the USA, for example, POP remains the most frequent indication for hysterectomy in women over 55 years of age [3]. In the light of the suggestions of Bonney and Nichols, it is timely that the urogynaecologic community revisit the surgical concept of "Why and when is it necessary or indicated to perform a hysterectomy at POP repair?" also considering the current female population, its living habits and the life expectation.

Determination of the best surgical treatment options involves consideration of a patient's values and preferences for uterine preservation vs. hysterectomy.

Based on the available urogynaecologic literature, there is no data to favour either removal or preservation of the uterus in women with POP; in fact, for example, in many studies, the comparison between hysterectomy with suspension of the

M. Serati, M.D. (✉)
Urogynecology Unit, Department of Obstetrics and Gynecology, University of Insubria, Varese, Italy

P. Sorice
Department of Obstetrics and Gynecology, Fornaroli Hospital, Magenta, Italy

© Springer International Publishing AG, part of Springer Nature 2018 145
V. Li Marzi, M. Serati (eds.), *Management of Pelvic Organ Prolapse*,
Urodynamics, Neurourology and Pelvic Floor Dysfunctions,
https://doi.org/10.1007/978-3-319-59195-7_12

uterosacral ligaments and sacrospinous hysteropexy does not differ at 12 months for anatomical recurrences, surgical complications and quality of life [4, 5].

Furthermore, the findings that hysterectomy may contribute to a higher success rate and to the development of urinary incontinence and/or female sexual dysfunction are not supported by evidence. It is not clear why both hysteropexy was sometimes performed in the presence of overt uterine prolapse and/or concomitant vaginal hysterectomy was often included in vaginal prolapse repair in the absence of uterine prolapse. In our opinion, it makes both anatomical and clinical sense to remove the uterus only (and always) when the uterus is one of the pelvic organs directly involved in the prolapse but to preserve and suspend the uterus otherwise.

To answer the question, we have to consider two different scenarios:

1. When the uterus is directly involved in the prolapse
2. When the uterus is not directly involved in the prolapse

12.1 When the Uterus Is Directly Involved in the Prolapse

It seems obvious that when the uterus is significantly prolapsed with evident loss of integrity of the uterosacral-cardinal ligament complex, then hysterectomy is a rational surgical option. However, several uterus-sparing procedures have been proposed in the literature as an alternative intervention in these cases like open or laparoscopic sacral hysteropexy, high uterosacral suspension, sacrospinous fixation, posterior IVS, etc.

The reasons given to preserve the uterus were:

1. Continuation of childbearing potential
2. Reduced risk of POP recurrence by keeping the uterus and its adjoining supportive structures in situ
3. Decreased sexual satisfaction after removal of the uterus
4. Increased long-term morbidity associated with hysterectomy, in particular new onset urinary incontinence
5. Higher rate of postoperative complications, including vaginal erosion, with hysterectomy but only in case of use of mesh to repair the vaginal prolapse
6. Natural menopausal timing
7. Less invasive and reduction surgical time and blood loss
8. Patience preference

The evidence in favour of these arguments is, however, poor:

1. Conservative management of uterovaginal prolapse (observation, pessary or pelvic floor physical therapy) should be the first-line treatment for women with uterovaginal prolapse who plan to attempt pregnancy.
2. POP surgery is performed in only a minute proportion of women in their reproductive age, and therefore, pregnancies reported after POP repair are extremely

rare. In the largest series of pregnancies after hysteropexy, only three women conceived spontaneously after the procedure and all three pregnancies were terminated [6].

3. There is no clear evidence regarding the role of uterine preservation in reducing the POP recurrence rate. In the majority of studies, the postoperative recurrence rates after hysterectomy compared to hysteropexy were similar, but the latter was associated with an earlier recovery [7].

4. The importance of the uterus, particularly the cervix, in female sexual function was largely discussed in the 1980s. It was proposed that the presence of the cervix could improve the quality of female orgasm and that hysterectomy (particularly vaginal hysterectomy) could damage the innervation and vascularization of the vagina and other orgasmic structures. There is no scientific data, however, to support this assumption. In contrast, most studies showed that removal of a non-healthy uterus (POP included) actually improves the female sexual function [8]. A recent report further showed that female sexual function does not get worse after hysterectomy for POP [9].

5. A large observational study suggested a significantly higher rate of urinary anti-incontinence surgery in women who previously underwent hysterectomy [10]. However, the correlation was not found after adjusting for a number of confounding variables particularly number of vaginal births. In another study comparing the effects of hysterectomy in identical twin pairs, hysterectomy and urinary incontinence were not related [11].

6. Many surgical series have shown that partial preservation of the uterus at laparoscopic repair of POP using mesh significantly reduces the risk of vaginal mesh erosions. This finding, however, will only apply in case of use of mesh and if the laparoscopic approach is selected for POP repair [12].

7. Even in women who undergo ovarian-sparing hysterectomies, ovarian function is affected. Two studies have compared ovarian function after ovarian-sparing hysterectomies with a nonsurgical control group. In these studies, menopause was defined as follicle-stimulating hormone levels of 40 IU/L or higher. In these cohorts, approximately twice as many women who underwent hysterectomy became menopausal during the 4–5-year study period.

8. Uterine preservation at the time of prolapse repair avoids an unnecessary procedure and has been associated with faster operative times and less blood loss and short hospitalization.

9. Frick et al. found that 60% of women indicated they would decline a hysterectomy if presented with an equally efficacious alternative to a hysterectomy-based prolapse repair. Those patients who were considered active decision makers and those who had family or friends who had negative experiences with hysterectomy were more likely to decline hysterectomy [13].

Similarly, Korbly et al. found that 36% of women preferred uterine preservation when presented with equally efficacious surgical options. Interestingly, 21% of women in this study continued to prefer uterine preservation, even when the uterine-sparing prolapse procedure was associated with worse efficacy. Patient preferences were associated with geographic region, with more patients in the West and Northeast favouring uterine conservation [14].

Preserving uterus has some limited disadvantages like risk of unanticipated uterine pathology.

In spite of this, the risk of cervical carcinoma has not been studied in hysteropexy, but data from studies evaluating supracervical hysterectomy can be extrapolated to uterine-sparing surgery. Even in studies that predated modern cytological and viral screening techniques, the rate of cervical carcinoma was low (below 0.3%).

With improved cytological and viral screening and the HPV vaccine, the true rate is likely to be even lower.

Studies evaluating uterine pathology also demonstrate low risks for endometrial hyperplasia and cancer. Currently, a noninvasive, cost-effective screening strategy does not exist for asymptomatic women desiring uterine-sparing surgery. Beyond a careful history, physical examination, Papanicolaou smear and HPV screening, there are not sufficient data to recommend routine screening for endometrial pathology. But there are some contraindications to preserve uterus although there is a prolapse concomitant like postmenopausal bleeding, tamoxifen therapy, familial cancer syndrome BRCA1–2, current or recent cervical dysplasia, etc.

12.2   When the Uterus Is Not Directly Involved in POP

Hysterectomy (or less frequently hysteropexy) is traditionally performed to repair apical compartment prolapse as well as mild uterine descensus according to the "tent theory" of Baden and Walker. In 1992, they mentioned that "we believe the first step in any anterior or posterior vaginal repair is to ensure grade 0 support at superior segmental and cul-de-sac sites" [15]. DeLancey's group subsequently demonstrated using quantitative dynamic MRI analysis that approximately half the degree of bladder displacement is associated with some degree of downward uterine displacement [16]. This observation clearly indicated that mild cases of anterior compartment prolapse does not require concomitant apical repair. In fact, Huffaker et al. reported that a careful repair of the anterior compartment with an adequate transverse cystocele repair is able to offer a very high objective and subjective cure rate of POP in cases of moderate uterine prolapse (stage II) without performing a large apical suspension [17]. Madhu et al. investigated the use of cervical traction under anaesthesia to measure the "real" stage of uterine prolapse in women with anterior vaginal descensus and mild uterine prolapse [18]. They found that preoperative cervical traction is not necessary as only anterior fascial repair with adequate transverse cystocele repair resulted in high postoperative cure rates of POP irrespective of the effect of "forced" uterine descensus.

Conclusion

Based on the available urogynaecologic literature, the role of hysterectomy in the surgical strategy of POP repair remains controversial. Currently, there is no data to favour either removal or preservation of the uterus in women with POP. Between the various surgical vaginal techniques of preserving the uterus, sacrospinous hysteropexy is the best studied. Quality of life and sexual function outcomes appear favourable after sacrospinous hysteropexy. Additionally, the sacrohysteropexy has been shown to have promising outcomes with results comparable with hysterectomy and sacrocolpopexy [19].

The findings that hysterectomy may contribute to a higher success rate and to the development of urinary incontinence and/or female sexual dysfunction are not supported by evidence. It is not clear why hysteropexy is sometimes performed in the presence of overt uterine prolapse. Likewise, it is not clear why a concomitant vaginal hysterectomy is often included in vaginal prolapse repair also in the absence of uterine prolapse. Before, it is important to select patients carefully for uterus-sparing prolapse repairs. Therefore, it makes both anatomical and clinical sense to remove the uterus only (and always) when the uterus is one of the pelvic organs directly involved in the prolapse but to preserve and suspend the uterus otherwise.

References

1. Maher C, Baessler K, Barber M, et al. Pelvic organ prolapse surgery. In: Abrams P, Cardozo L, Khoury S, Wein A, editors. 5th International Consultation on Incontinence. Paris: Health Publication Ltd; 2013. p. 1393.
2. Nichols DH. What is new in vaginal surgery? Int Urogynecol J Pelvic Floor Dysfunct. 1996;7:115–6.
3. Baggish MS. Total and subtotal abdominal hysterectomy. Best Pract Res Clin Obstet Gynaecol. 2005;19:333–56.
4. Detollenaere RJ, den Boon J, Stekelenburg J, IntHout J, Vierhout ME, Kluivers KB, van Eijndhoven HWF. Sacrospinous hysteropexy versus vaginal hysterectomy with suspension of the uterosacral ligaments in women with uterine prolapse stage 2 or higher: multicentre randomised non-inferiority trial. BMJ. 2015;351:h3717.
5. Maher CF, Cary MP, Slack MC, Murray CJ, Milligan M, Schluter P. Uterine preservation or hysterectomy at sacrospinous colpopexy for uterovaginal prolapse. Int Urogynecol J Pelvic Floor Dysfunct. 2001;12(6):381–4. (Discussion 4–5. PubMed Epub 2002/01/25.eng).
6. Barranger E, Fritel X, Pigne A. Abdominal sacrohysteropexy in young women with uterovaginal prolapse: long-term follow-up. Am J Obstet Gynecol. 2003;189:1245–50.
7. Dietz V, Schraffordt Koops SE, van der Vaart CH. Vaginal surgery for uterine descent; which options do we have? A review of the literature. Int Urogynecol J Pelvic Floor Dysfunct. 2009;20:349–56.
8. Rhodes JC, Kjerulff KH, Langenberg PW, Guzinski GM. Hysterectomy and sexual functioning. JAMA. 1999;282:1934–41.
9. Zucchi A, Costantini E, Mearini L, Fioretti F, Bini V, Porena M. Female sexual dysfunction in urogenital prolapse surgery: colposacropexy vs. hysterocolposacropexy. J Sex Med. 2008;5:139–45.
10. Altman D, Granath F, Cnattingius S, Falconer C. Hysterectomy and risk of stress-urinary-incontinence surgery: nationwide cohort study. Lancet. 2007;370:1494–9.
11. Miller JJ, Botros SM, Beaumont JL, et al. Impact of hysterectomy on stress urinary incontinence: an identical twin study. Am J Obstet Gynecol. 2008;198(565):e1–4.
12. Collinet P, Belot F, Debodinance P, Ha Duc E, Lucot JP, Cosson M. Transvaginal mesh technique for pelvic organ prolapse repair: mesh exposure management and risk factors. Int Urogynecol J Pelvic Floor Dysfunct. 2006;17:315–20.

13. Frick AC, Barber MD, Paraiso MF, Ridgeway B, Jelovsek JE, Walters MD. Attitudes toward hysterectomy in women undergoing evaluation for uterovaginal prolapse. Female Pelvic Med Reconstr Surg. 2013;19:103–9.
14. Korbly NB, Kassis NC, Good MM, et al. Patient preferences for uterine preservation and hysterectomy in women with pelvic organ prolapse. Am J Obstet Gynecol. 2013;209:470.e1–6.
15. Baden WF, Walker T. Surgical repair of vaginal defects. Philadelphia: Lippincott Williams & Wilkins; 1992.
16. Summers A, Winkel LA, Hussain HK, DeLancey JO. The relationship between anterior and apical compartment support. Am J Obstet Gynecol. 2006;194:1438–43.
17. Huffaker RK, Kuehl TJ, Muir TW, Yandell PM, Pierce LM, Shull BL. Transverse cystocele repair with uterine preservation using native tissue. Int Urogynecol J Pelvic Floor Dysfunct. 2008;19:1275–81.
18. Madhu C, Foon R, Agur W, Smith P. Does traction on the cervix under anaesthesia tell us when to perform a concomitant hysterectomy? A 2-year follow-up of a prospective cohort study. Int Urogynecol J Pelvic Floor Dysfunct. 2014;25:1213–7.
19. Ridgeway BM. Does prolapse equal hysterectomy? The role of uterine conservation in women with uterovaginal prolapse. Am J Obstet Gynecol. 2015;213(6):802–9.

Part IV

Outcome and Follow-up

Prolapse Surgery and Outcome Measures

13

Rhiannon Bray and Alex Digesu

13.1 Introduction

A number of outcome measures can be used when considering the surgical treatment of pelvic organ prolapse (POP).

In 2010 the International Continence Society (ICS) reviewed 32 articles, which had a primary focus on surgical treatment of prolapse to assess the status of outcome measure reporting [1]. According to Oxford levels of evidence, only 12/32 were level 1, 2 or 3, while 17 were graded as level 4. Symptoms were characterised in 27/32 (84%), but standardised symptom questionnaires were sporadically used. Urinary symptoms were reported in 20/32 (63%), faecal symptoms in 8/32 (25%) and both urinary and faecal symptoms in 7/32 (22%). Sexual function was reported in 16 of 32 articles (50%). All studies used some outcome measure as a gauge of anatomical success. Ten of 32 articles (31%) used the pelvic organ prolapse quantification (POP-Q) system. Five of 32 (16%) used a modified Baden-Walker scale, and the remainder used some other method. In 6 of 32 articles (19%), quality of life data were available, at least in a limited form. Complications were reported in 29 of 32 (90%) studies, and no articles gave significant socioeconomic data, with only 4 of 32 (13%) reporting on length of stay data.

A recent joint report from the ICS and International Urogynecological Association [IUGA] recommended that the following outcomes should be reported in studies of POP surgery: objective outcomes (e.g. POP-Q), patient-reported outcomes (particularly the presence or absence of vaginal bulge symptoms), satisfaction outcomes, quality of life (QoL) and perioperative data (e.g. operative time, hospital stay, etc.) [2].

R. Bray · A. Digesu (✉)
Imperial College NHS Trust, London, UK
e-mail: a.digesu@imperial.ac.uk

© Springer International Publishing AG, part of Springer Nature 2018
V. Li Marzi, M. Serati (eds.), *Management of Pelvic Organ Prolapse*,
Urodynamics, Neurourology and Pelvic Floor Dysfunctions,
https://doi.org/10.1007/978-3-319-59195-7_13

13.2   Patient-Reported Outcomes: Quality of Life

POP can have detrimental effects on women's QoL. Vaginal, urinary, bowel and sexual dysfunction often coexists and can impact upon the patient's daily life causing physical, social, personal limitations, depression and low self-esteem. Accordingly, for an individual patient, the most important outcome of a surgical procedure is the relief of her symptoms and improvement in her quality of life [3].

Currently the only valid tools available to assess the patient-reported outcomes are psychometrically robust questionnaires, and as such their use has been recommended and advocated by ICS, IUGA, the National Institutes of Health (NIH) and the International Consultation on Incontinence (ICI) [1, 4–10]. Accordingly, in the last decade, their use has increased in both clinical and research practice, and they are now widely employed to measure the impact of POP surgery on women's quality of life and patient satisfaction. This has even lead to the suggestion that QoL should be considered as an end point in all clinical trials [11].

The range of questionnaires available for POP is much less than those for urinary incontinence, and few questionnaires on vaginal and pelvic floor problems are considered as highly recommended. In 2005 the Symptom and Quality of Life Committee of the ICI performed a systematic review of questionnaires related to urinary/anal incontinence and vaginal and pelvic floor problems and concluded that 18 questionnaires achieved grade A status in the assessment of urinary incontinence, whereas in the area of anal incontinence and vaginal and pelvic floor problems, only two of the questionnaires could be considered grade B and five grade C [1].

The clinician's choice of tool should be guided by the particular outcome they would like to measure as well as based on the instrument they are more familiar with. It is also important to remember that administering too many questionnaires to a patient may not be helpful as patient's fatigue can lead to erroneous answers. Long forms of questionnaires may be desirable for research studies where detail is needed, while short forms may have wider applicability in clinical practice where it is important to minimise respondent burden and cost. It is generally desirable to use a validated, simple, self-completed, psychometrically robust, easy to understand and complete questionnaire that is widely accepted and has been previously used in the targeted population [10].

There are a number of validated questionnaires available for this purpose; however, their ability to detect changes can vary [10]. They include symptom and QoL scales specific for urinary function and pelvic disorder colorectal function, as well as more generic instruments that measure general and social and emotional wellbeing. The majority of these have been assessed for validity and reliability, are fairly lengthy, cover a range of symptoms and include a number of subscales related to urinary and bowel disorders.

It is also recommended that the sexual function status of all individual participant's pre- and post-intervention should be reported [1]. Some condition-specific questionnaires incorporate assessment of sexual function [8], but specific validated questionnaires on sexual function are also available and provide a discreet and reproducible method for evaluating sexual health. The Pelvic Organ Prolapse/

Incontinence Sexual Questionnaire [PISQ] [12] and the Female Sexual Function Index [FSFI] [13] are two questionnaires most frequently used.

13.3   Patient-Reported Outcome Measures: Symptoms

POP is frequently associated with urinary and faecal symptoms. In a study of over 200 women with POP, 73% had concomitant urinary incontinence, 86% had urinary urgency and/or frequency, 34–62% complained of voiding dysfunction, and 31% experienced faecal incontinence [14].

The single most consistent symptom associated with POP appears to be the presence of a vaginal 'lump' or 'bulge' [5, 14–17]. In fact the presence of this symptom can be reliably correlated with the anatomical severity of the prolapse. Prolapse that extends beyond the hymen is associated with a greater sensation of a 'lump' and worse symptoms [5, 14–17]. Postoperative resolution of bulge symptoms is associated with greater improvements in QoL, compared to anatomical improvements [3].

Studies have shown that POP surgery can improve other pelvic floor symptoms. In a study by Fayyad et al., increased urinary frequency, urgency, poor urinary stream and incomplete bladder emptying improved significantly after anterior and posterior repair; urge incontinence improved with anterior repair but not with posterior repair. Stress urinary incontinence did not improve after anterior or posterior repair, and bowel symptoms improved after posterior repair [18].

13.4   Individual Questionnaires

13.4.1 Pelvic Floor Distress Inventory (PFDI) and Pelvic Floor Impact Questionnaire (PFIQ)

The *Pelvic Floor Distress Inventory* (PFDI) and *Pelvic Floor Impact Questionnaire* (PFIQ) were developed in 2001 by Barber et al. [5, 6]. The PFDI was designed to evaluate the symptom distress or bother in women with pelvic floor dysfunction. It is an expansion of the *Urogenital Distress Inventory* (UDI); it includes all the items of the original UDI questionnaire and has additional questions related to POP and colorectal dysfunction (26). It encompasses 46 items divided into three domains: (1) UDI (28 items), (2) Colorectal-Anal Distress Inventory (17 items) and (3) Pelvic Organ Prolapse Distress Inventory (16 items).

The PFIQ was designed to assess the impact of the pelvic floor disorders on women's life. Similarly it was an expansion of a previous questionnaire, the *Incontinence Impact Questionnaire* (IIQ) [19]. It contains all the items included in the original IIQ and has additional items related to other pelvic floor dysfunction. It has 93 items divided in three domains: (1) Urinary Impact Questionnaire (UIQ), (2) Pelvic Organ Prolapse Impact Questionnaire (POPIQ) and (3) Colorectal-Anal Impact Questionnaire (CRAIQ).

PFDI and PFIQ have shown good validity and reliability (both content and construct). However their use in clinical practice has been restricted as they are time consuming, taking roughly 23 min to complete. In order to combat this, the authors developed and validated abridged versions [20]. The PFDI-20 contains 20 items instead of 46, and the PFIQ-7 includes 7 items instead of 93. They are particularly useful when evaluating the outcomes of therapy that may take some time to show clinical benefit as they have a 3-month recall period [5, 6]. To date these questionnaires have been translated in Korean, Spanish, Greek, Danish, Turkish, Swedish and French [21–29].

13.4.2 Prolapse Quality of Life (P-QoL)

The prolapse quality of life (P-QoL) questionnaire was developed in 2004 by Digesu et al. in order to provide a shorter comprehensive tool able to investigate both the severity of POP symptoms and their impact on women's QoL [4]. The P-QoL is considered a valid, reliable self-completed questionnaire which is easy to understand and to complete. Individual domain scores are significantly different between symptomatic and asymptomatic women (good content reliability) and significantly higher in women with more advanced/severe POP stages (good construct reliability). It contains 20 questions divided into nine domains: general health (1 item), prolapse impact (1 item), role (2 items), physical (2 items) and social limitations (3 items), personal relationships (2 items), emotional limitations (3 items), sleep/ energy disturbance (2 items) and severity measurement (4 items). Responses are according to a four-point Likert Scale: 'none/not at all', 'slightly/a little', 'moderately' and 'a lot'. A score is calculated for each domain ranging from 0 to 100. A higher score indicates a greater impairment of QoL or poor QoL. In addition to the QoL items, the P-QoL also includes 18 symptom questions: 11 urogenital (bladder, sexual) and 7 bowel. The responses are categorised using the same scale plus an additional 'not applicable' option if the women do not have the symptom. These symptom's questions are not used to provide any scoring.

To date the P-QoL has been translated and validated in several languages including English, Italian, Dutch, Thai, Slovakian, Portuguese, German, Turkish, Persian, Japanese, Spanish and French and used in clinical as well as research practice [4, 30–38].

13.4.3 Pelvic Floor Dysfunction Questionnaire

The Pelvic Floor Dysfunction Questionnaire (PFDQ) was designed by Ellerkmann et al. in 2001 and can be used to correlate the location and severity of prolapse with the associated pelvic floor symptoms [14]. Again this questionnaire has 65 questions that were assembled from commonly used validated instruments. The PFDQ encompasses eight domains, each relating to a specific type of dysfunction. The domains are urinary incontinence, irritative urinary symptoms, voiding dysfunction, POP symptoms, faecal incontinence, defaecatory dysfunction, pelvic pain and sexual dysfunction. Again a Likert scale is used to quantify the severity, the duration of symptoms and the impact on QoL.

The validity and reliability of this questionnaire have never been tested. However, the authors did test this questionnaire on 237 women and concluded that POP symptoms do not necessarily correlate with compartment-specific defects and increasing severity of POP is weakly to moderately associated to urinary, defaecatory and sexual dysfunction [14].

13.4.4 Danish Prolapse Questionnaire

The Danish Prolapse Questionnaire was developed and validated by Mouritsen et al. in 2003. Like the PFDI, it is used to evaluate the symptom distress in women with POP [39]. It contains 34 questions divided into four domains: (1) mechanical symptoms, (2) lower urinary tract symptoms (LUTS), (3) bowel symptoms and (4) sexual symptoms. The severity of each symptom is graded according to how often it is experienced (1, never or less than once/month; 2, less than once/week; 3, once or more/week; 4, daily). An additional four-point bother score assesses how each symptom affects QoL. Again the psychometric properties (validity and reliability) of this questionnaire have not been tested yet.

13.4.5 ICIQ-Vaginal Symptoms Questionnaire

The ICIQ-Vaginal Symptoms questionnaire was developed and validated by Price et al. in 2006 [7]. It was designed to assess the severity of POP symptoms (both vaginal and sexual), to measure their impact on QoL and importantly to evaluate the treatment outcomes. ICIQ-VS is self-administered and has 14 individual items. It has shown a high internal consistency (Cronbach's alpha 0.70 and 0.84 for vaginal and sexual symptoms, respectively) and a good sensitivity to change. It is particularly useful as it is a simple, reliable, valid tool, able to measure the severity of vaginal and sexual symptoms in women with POP as well as evaluating their impact on QoL.

13.4.6 Australian Pelvic Floor Questionnaire

The Australian Pelvic Floor Questionnaire can be used as a self- and/or interviewer-completed questionnaire. Questions are distributed between four domains: bladder function (15 items), bowel function (12 items), prolapse symptoms (5 items) and sexual function (10 items). A four-point scoring system is used to assess the frequency, severity, and bother of pelvic floor symptoms for the majority of the items. The score for each of the four domains ranges between 0 and 10. The maximum total pelvic floor dysfunction score is 40 or 30 if a woman is not sexually active.

Both the self- and interviewer-completed questionnaires have been proved to be simple, easy to complete, valid, reliable and sensitive to change [8, 40].

13.4.7 Pelvic Organ Prolapse/Urinary Incontinence Sexual Questionnaire (PISQ)

The Pelvic Organ Prolapse/Urinary Incontinence Sexual Questionnaire (PISQ) was designed to assess sexual function in women with POP and/or urinary incontinence [41]. It encompasses 31 items divided into three domains: (1) behavioural/ emotive (15 items), (2) physical (10 items) and (3) partner- related (6 items). Responses are graded on a five-point Likert scale from 'never' to 'always'. PISQ was validated in two phases. In phase 1, PISQ scores from 83 women were correlated with Incontinence Impact Questionnaire-7 (IIQ-7) scores. In phase 2, the PISQ scores from 99 women were compared with the Sexual History Form-12 (SHF-12). As there was a high correlation between the domain scores of the PISQ and the previously validated IIQ-7 and SHF-12 scores, the authors concluded that PISQ is a valid, reliable and useful instrument for the assessment of women with POP. A short form of this questionnaire has also been developed and validated (PSIQ-12) [42].

13.4.8 The Electronic Personal Assessment-Pelvic Floor (ePAQ-PF)

The ePAQ-PF questionnaire was developed as a valid instrument to evaluate the impact of urinary, bowel, vaginal and sexual symptoms on QoL. It also includes additional domains on dyspareunia and general sex life. The questionnaire employs a novel computer-based interview process and was developed from three pre-existing questionnaires: the Birmingham Bowel and Urinary Symptoms Questionnaire (BBUSQ-22) [43], the Sheffield Prolapse Symptoms Questionnaire (SPSQ) [44] and the Female Sexual Function Index (FSFI) questionnaire [13].

The BBUSQ-22 is a 22-item questionnaire developed to assess patients with functional bowel and urinary symptoms. The SPSQ specifically assesses symptom severity in women with anatomical and functional pelvic floor disorders. It is divided in four domains: (1) lump and pain, (2) bladder function, (3) bowel function and (4) sexual function. It also includes a final evaluation of the impact of POP symptoms on woman's QoL. The FSFI is a validated 19-item questionnaire, developed as a multidimensional tool to evaluate female sexual function. It provides scores on six domains of sexual function (desire, arousal, lubrication, orgasm, satisfaction and pain) as well as a total score.

ePAQ-PF has four domains (urinary 35 items, bowel 33 items, vaginal 22 items and sexual 28 items). All items score between 0 and 3 (0 indicating best and 3 indicating worst health status). These domain scores are calculated by dividing the sum of all items in the domain by the total possible item score and multiplying this by 100, to produce a scale 0 to 100. The higher the score, the worst possible health status. The 'bother' associated with a particular symptom is scored using a four-point scale (0 = not a problem, 1 = a bit of a problem, 2 = quite a problem and 3 = a serious problem).

In order to assess the validity and reliability of this study, a cross-sectional study of 599 women with pelvic floor disorders was undertaken. Internal reliability, levels of missing data, secondary factor analysis, floor and ceiling effects, descriptive statistics, item-to-total correlation scores, item discriminant and convergent validity were measured. All 19 domains were internally reliable with Cronbach's alpha scores ranging from 0.71 to 0.93. Missing response rates ranged from 0.2 to 1.3%. All items were found to be most highly correlated with their own corrected scale. Therefore the authors concluded that the ePAQ-PF is a valid and reliable instrument to assess (1) the severity and bother of pelvic floor disorders, (2) the impact of pelvic floor disorders on women's QoL and (3) the treatment outcome [45, 46].

The particular advantages of this computerised instrument are the reduction of missing data and the high satisfaction ratings, probably due to the greater privacy enabled by this type of administration. Of particular use is the fact that ePAQ allows the direct imputation of the responses into a database. However, the cost of technology required and the importance of patient's computer literacy may prove to limit the widespread applicability of this particular tool especially considering that the majority of women with POP are elderly.

13.4.9 Patient Global Impression of Improvement (PGI-I): Satisfaction/Symptoms

The Patient Global Impression of Improvement (PGI-I) is a seven-point scale that is a simple, direct, easy to use scale that can be used in both clinical and research practice. It was derived from the Clinical Global Impression-Improvement scale. It is a scale that requires the patient to assess how much the illness has improved or worsened relative baseline. It has been validated for use in female patients following intervention for both urinary incontinence and prolapse [47, 48]. It has also been demonstrated to have excellent test-retest reliability [48]. The stem of the questionnaire has also been modified for use in patients with stress urinary incontinence but maintaining the response options [47].

13.4.10 Visual Analogue Scale: Satisfaction/Symptoms

Visual Analogue Scale (VAS) uses a 10 cm line, and responders are asked to mark the severity of their symptom somewhere along the line. 0 indicates no complains and 10 is the maximum. It was originally developed for the assessment of pain but can be reproducibly be used to indicate severity of symptoms or bother. Urogynaecologists have made use of the quick and simple nature of this tool in clinical practice to investigate pelvic floor disorder symptoms as well as treatment satisfaction and outcome. This scale has been shown to be valid, repeatable, and simple to use. VAS bother scores of 636 women were significantly associated with both clinical and ultrasound measures of POP [49].

13.4.11 Pelvic Organ Prolapse Symptom Score (POP-SS): Symptoms

The pelvic organ prolapse symptom score (POP-SS) is a useful tool to assess treatment effectiveness. It includes a set of questions on the symptoms caused or exacerbated specifically by POP. It was designed and validated in 2008 by Hagen who proposed its use to assess POP symptoms before and after treatment, as well as its use in randomised controlled trials of various interventions for POP [50]. POP-SS has been evaluated in three patient groups: postpartum women, patient who have undergone pelvic floor muscle training and those undergoing surgical repair of POP. It has good internal consistency (Cronbach's alpha 0.723–0.823), has good construct reliability and is sensitive to change [51]. It consists of seven items, each with a five-point Likert response (0 = never, 4 = all the time). A total score (0–28) is calculated by adding the seven responses. There is also an additional question to identify the particular symptoms which causes the most bother.

13.5 Objective Outcome Measures: Anatomy

ICS recommends that a standard, validated and reliable method of describing subjects anatomy, such as the POP-Q, should be used before and after surgical intervention [1]. This system was introduced by Bump in 1996 and uses the relationship between six anatomical points in various segments of the vagina, and a fixed reference point, the hymen, to stage POP. Staging ranges between good support (POP-Q stage 0 or 1) and complete lack of support (POP-Q stage 4) [9].

Despite this tool has greatly improved reliability in the assessment of anatomical success in POP surgeries, the objective outcome measures in POP surgery in general have been questioned [52]. Over 75% of women who attend for annual gynaecological examinations and who do not report symptoms of prolapse will have POP-Q stage greater than 1, and 40% have POP-Q stage 2 or greater prolapse. According to the current NIH criteria, these women would be defined as 'surgical failures', but these findings appear to fall within the normal distribution of vaginal support for parous women [53, 54]. More recent work has focused on the hymen and proposed that anatomical failure after surgery is defined a POP that extends beyond this point [3, 55–58].

Questions have been raised regarding the ability of the system to describe in sufficient detail the individual measurements of POP-Q and discriminate between clinically important groups, such as stage 2 or 3 [52]. It is also not clear if apical prolapse should be staged in the same fashion as anterior or posterior wall prolapse. The impact of observer bias should also be considered when considering surgical outcomes. Retrospective reports of cystocele repair success rate range from 80 to 100% [59–62], whereas prospective studies give lower rates of 37–67% [63, 64]. Blinding of the assessor in randomised controlled trials has been shown to lead to increased recurrence rates at 3 months and 1 year versus an unblinded assessor [65]. A particular controversy highlighted by the ICI is the increasing trend for authors with financial conflicts of interest related to the commercial products being evaluated reporting the outcomes of surgical interventions, which further increases the risk of reporting bias [52].

13.5.1   FIGO Assessment Scoring System (FASS)

Digesu et al. on behalf of the International Federation of Gynaecology and Obstetrics (FIGO) Working Group on Pelvic Floor Dysfunction developed the FIGO assessment scoring system (FASS). It was designed to be a very simplistic holistic tool that incorporates the anatomic examination findings (P); the associated functional disorders such as bladder, bowel as well as prolapse symptoms (S); and the severity and degree of symptom bother (B) similarly to the tumour (T), nodes (N) and metastases' (M) system for gynaecological malignancy. This scoring system is intended for use by a wide range of clinicians in the evaluation of women with pelvic floor dysfunction. The system was designed to be very simplistic so that it may be adopted by a wide range of clinicians who provide women's health care at facilities with low resources.

The FIGO assessment scoring system for pelvic floor dysfunction has passed the test to examine its interobserver and intraobserver correlation. In addition, it has documented construct validity in that subjects with complaints of pelvic floor dysfunction had higher scores then subjects without pelvic floor disorders [66].

13.6   Objective Outcome Measures: Reoperation Rate

Reoperation rate can also be used to measure the outcome of surgery, but it must be understood that a large number of reoperations may be lost to follow-up and numbers seen may be an underestimation. Another particular controversy relates to same versus different compartment reoperations. Rates as high as 30% have been reported by large studies. However this is bias by the lack of differentiation between operations for POP and those for stress incontinence or whether or not the repeated surgery was in the same or a different vaginal compartment [67]. When considering site-specific recurrence, much lower rates of 3.4–9.7% are quoted [68, 69]. These discrepancies have led to IUGA/ICS issuing standardised terminology [1] (see Table 13.1).

Table 13.1 IUGA/ICS standardised terminology on definitions of reoperation

Primary surgery: first procedure required for the treatment of POP in any compartment
Further surgery: this gives a global figure for the number of subsequent procedures the patient undergoes directly or indirectly relating to the primary surgery. This is subdivided into:
(a) *Primary prolapse surgery/different site*. A prolapse procedure in a new site/compartment following previous surgery in a different compartment (e.g. anterior repair following previous posterior repair)
(b) *Repeat surgery is a repeat operation for prolapse arising from the same site*. Where combinations of procedures arise, e.g. new anterior repair plus further posterior repair, these should be reported separately, i.e. repeat posterior repair and primary anterior repair
(c) *Surgery for complications*: e.g. mesh exposure or extrusion or pain or patient compromise, e.g. haemorrhage
(d) *Surgery for non-prolapse-related conditions*: e.g. subsequent surgery for stress urinary incontinence or faecal incontinence

13.7   Defining Treatment Success

Despite the NIH workshop definition of 'satisfactory anatomic outcome' (POP-Q stage 0 or 1), wide variability of the definition of success still exists. Using the NIH definition, 'success' rates as low as 30% have been reported in the literature [64, 70]. Because of this, other groups have chosen to use the Baden-Walker classification system or the combination of anatomical outcome and symptoms [70–74]. This variability makes it difficult to compare successful outcomes across studies [75–77].

This point is well illustrated in the secondary analysis of the Colpopexy and Urinary Reduction Efforts (CARE) trial [3].Using a combination of anatomical, symptom and retreatment outcomes, 18 different definitions of success were applied to the data. 'Success' ranged between 19.2 and 97.2%. It was highest if the absence of retreatment was considered 'success' and lowest when anatomical parameters alone were used. Again the absence of 'bulge' symptoms was closely linked to the perceived 'success' of the surgery and overall improvement. This leads to the NIH Pelvic Floor Disorders Network recommendations that (1) any definition of success after POP surgery should include the absence of bulge symptoms in addition to anatomic criteria and the absence of retreatment and (2) using the hymen as a threshold for anatomic success seems a reasonable and defensible approach [3]. The ICI recommends that subjective success postoperatively should be defined as the absence of vaginal bulge (Grade C) [52].

Conclusion

Defining the 'success' of POP treatment is not as simple as it seems. Historically, the majority of authors focused exclusively on anatomical success ignoring other important areas such as the presence, absence and severity of associated symptoms, sexual function, QoL and patient's satisfaction. When considering outcome measures, all of the above should be considered. To the patient herself, the most important outcome is the relief of her symptoms and improvement of her QoL [3]. Therefore, in the recent years, more attention has been paid to the complex relationships between POP and its often coexisting symptoms as well as on the impact of POP on women's QoL.

References

1. Brubaker L, et al. Surgery for pelvic organ prolapse. Female Pelvic Med Reconstr Surg. 2010;16(1):9–19.
2. Toozs-Hobson P, et al. An International Urogynecological Association (IUGA)/International Continence Society (ICS) joint report on the terminology for reporting outcomes of surgical procedures for pelvic organ prolapse. Neurourol Urodyn. 2012;31(4):415–21.
3. Barber MD, et al. Defining success after surgery for pelvic organ prolapse. Obstet Gynecol. 2009;114(3):600–9.
4. Digesu GA, et al. P-QoL: a validated questionnaire to assess the symptoms and quality of life of women with urogenital prolapse. Int Urogynecol J Pelvic Floor Dysfunct. 2005;16(3):176–81; discussion 181.

5. Barber MD, Walters MD, Bump RC. Short forms of two condition-specific quality-of-life questionnaires for women with pelvic floor disorders (PFDI-20 and PFIQ-7). Am J Obstet Gynecol. 2005;193(1):103–13.
6. Barber MD, et al. Psychometric evaluation of 2 comprehensive condition-specific quality of life instruments for women with pelvic floor disorders. Am J Obstet Gynecol. 2001;185(6):1388–95.
7. Price N, et al. Development and psychometric evaluation of the ICIQ Vaginal Symptoms Questionnaire: the ICIQ-VS. BJOG. 2006;113(6):700–12.
8. Baessler K, et al. A validated self-administered female pelvic floor questionnaire. Int Urogynecol J. 2010;21(2):163–72.
9. Bump RC, et al. The standardization of terminology of female pelvic organ prolapse and pelvic floor dysfunction. Am J Obstet Gynecol. 1996;175(1):10–7.
10. Parker-Autry CY, et al. Measuring outcomes in urogynecological surgery: "perspective is everything". Int Urogynecol J. 2013;24(1):15–25.
11. Glaser A, et al. Quality of life. Lancet. 1995;346(8972):444–5.
12. Rogers GR, et al. Sexual function in women with and without urinary incontinence and/or pelvic organ prolapse. Int Urogynecol J Pelvic Floor Dysfunct. 2001;12(6):361–5.
13. Rosen R, et al. The Female Sexual Function Index (FSFI): a multidimensional self-report instrument for the assessment of female sexual function. J Sex Marital Ther. 2000;26(2):191–208.
14. Ellerkmann RM, et al. Correlation of symptoms with location and severity of pelvic organ prolapse. Am J Obstet Gynecol. 2001;185(6):1332–7; discussion 1337-8.
15. Swift SE, Tate SB, Nicholas J. Correlation of symptoms with degree of pelvic organ support in a general population of women: what is pelvic organ prolapse? Am J Obstet Gynecol. 2003;189(2):372–7; discussion 377-9.
16. Bradley CS, Nygaard IE. Vaginal wall descensus and pelvic floor symptoms in older women. Obstet Gynecol. 2005;106(4):759–66.
17. Tan JS, et al. Predictive value of prolapse symptoms: a large database study. Int Urogynecol J Pelvic Floor Dysfunct. 2005;16(3):203–9; discussion 209.
18. Fayyad AM, et al. Symptomatic and quality of life outcomes after site-specific fascial reattachment for pelvic organ prolapse repair. Int Urogynecol J Pelvic Floor Dysfunct. 2008;19(2):191–7.
19. Nygaard I, et al. Prevalence of symptomatic pelvic floor disorders in US women. JAMA. 2008;300(11):1311–6.
20. Jelovsek JE, Maher C, Barber MD. Pelvic organ prolapse. Lancet. 2007;369(9566):1027–38.
21. Uebersax JS, et al. Short forms to assess life quality and symptom distress for urinary incontinence in women: the Incontinence Impact Questionnaire and the Urogenital Distress Inventory. Continence Program for Women Research Group. Neurourol Urodyn. 1995;14(2):131–9.
22. Kaplan PB, Sut N, Sut HK. Validation, cultural adaptation and responsiveness of two pelvic-floor-specific quality-of-life questionnaires, PFDI-20 and PFIQ-7, in a Turkish population. Eur J Obstet Gynecol Reprod Biol. 2012;162(2):229–33.
23. Yoo E-H, et al. Translation and linguistic validation of Korean version of short form of pelvic floor distress inventory-20, pelvic floor impact questionnaire-7. Obstet Gynecol Sci. 2013;56(5):330.
24. Sánchez-Sánchez B, et al. Cultural adaptation and validation of the Pelvic Floor Distress Inventory Short Form (PFDI-20) and Pelvic Floor Impact Questionnaire Short Form (PFIQ-7) Spanish versions. Eur J Obstet Gynecol Reprod Biol. 2013;170(1):281–5.
25. Grigoriadis T, et al. Translation and psychometric evaluation of the Greek short forms of two condition-specific quality of life questionnaires for women with pelvic floor disorders: PFDI-20 and PFIQ-7. Int Urogynecol J. 2013;24(12):2131–44.
26. Due U, Brostrøm S, Lose G. Validation of the Pelvic Floor Distress Inventory-20 and the pelvic floor impact questionnaire-7 in Danish women with pelvic organ prolapse. Acta Obstet Gynecol Scand. 2013;92(9):1041–8.
27. Toprak Celenay S, et al. Validity and reliability of the Turkish version of the Pelvic Floor Distress Inventory-20. Int Urogynecol J. 2012;23(8):1123–7.

28. Teleman PIA, et al. Validation of the Swedish short forms of the Pelvic Floor Impact Questionnaire (PFIQ-7), Pelvic Floor Distress Inventory (PFDI-20) and Pelvic Organ Prolapse/Urinary Incontinence Sexual Questionnaire (PISQ-12). Acta Obstet Gynecol Scand. 2011;90(5):483–7.
29. Omotosho TB, et al. Validation of Spanish versions of the Pelvic Floor Distress Inventory (PFDI) and Pelvic Floor Impact Questionnaire (PFIQ): a multicenter validation randomized study. Int Urogynecol J. 2009;20(6):623–39.
30. Svihrova V, et al. Validation of the Slovakian version of the P-QoL questionnaire. Int Urogynecol J. 2009;21(1):53–61.
31. de Tayrac R, et al. Validation linguistique en français des versions courtes des questionnaires de symptômes (PFDI-20) et de qualité de vie (PFIQ-7) chez les patientes présentant un trouble de la statique pelvienne. J Gynécol Obstét Biol Reprod. 2007;36(8):738–48.
32. Claerhout F, et al. Validity, reliability and responsiveness of a Dutch version of the prolapse quality-of-life (P-QoL) questionnaire. Int Urogynecol J. 2010;21(5):569–78.
33. Manchana T, Bunyavejchevin S. Validation of the Prolapse Quality of Life (P-QoL) questionnaire in Thai version. Int Urogynecol J. 2010;21(8):985–93.
34. de Oliveira MS, Tamanini JTN, de Aguiar Cavalcanti G. Validation of the Prolapse Quality-of-Life Questionnaire (P-QoL) in Portuguese version in Brazilian women. Int Urogynecol J. 2009;20(10):1191–202.
35. Lenz F, et al. Validation of a German version of the P-QoL Questionnaire. Int Urogynecol J. 2009;20(6):641–9.
36. Fukumoto Y, et al. Assessment of quality of life in women with pelvic organ prolapse: conditional translation and trial of P-QoL for use in Japan. Jpn H Urol. 2008;99(3):531–42.
37. Cam C, et al. Validation of the prolapse quality of life questionnaire (P-QoL) in a Turkish population. Eur J Obstet Gynecol Reprod Biol. 2007;135(1):132–5.
38. Digesu GA, et al. Validation of an Italian version of the prolapse quality of life questionnaire. Eur J Obstet Gynecol Reprod Biol. 2003;106(2):184–92.
39. Mouritsen L, Larsen JP. Symptoms, bother and POPQ in women referred with pelvic organ prolapse. Int Urogynecol J Pelvic Floor Dysfunct. 2003;14(2):122–7.
40. Baessler K, et al. Australian pelvic floor questionnaire: a validated interviewer-administered pelvic floor questionnaire for routine clinic and research. Int Urogynecol J Pelvic Floor Dysfunct. 2009;20(2):149–58.
41. Rogers RG, et al. A new instrument to measure sexual function in women with urinary incontinence or pelvic organ prolapse. Am J Obstet Gynecol. 2001;184(4):552–8.
42. Rogers RG, et al. A short form of the pelvic organ Prolapse/Urinary Incontinence Sexual Questionnaire (PISQ-12). Int Urogynecol Floor Dysfunct. 2003;14(3):164–8. Aug discussion 168 Epub Jul 25 Erratum in Int Urogynecol Floor Dysfunct MayJun153219, 2004. 14(3 SRC – GoogleScholar).
43. Hiller L, et al. Development and validation of a questionnaire for the assessment of bowel and lower urinary tract symptoms in women. BJOG. 2002;109(4):413–23.
44. Bradshaw HD, et al. Development and psychometric testing of a symptom index for pelvic organ prolapse. J Obstet Gynaecol. 2006;26(3):241–52.
45. Jones GL, et al. Responsiveness of the electronic Personal Assessment Questionnaire-Pelvic Floor (ePAQ-PF). Int Urogynecol J Pelvic Floor Dysfunct. 2009;20(5):557–64.
46. Ulrich D, et al. Use of a visual analog scale for evaluation of bother from pelvic organ prolapse. Ultrasound Obstet Gynecol. 2014;43(6):693–7.
47. Yalcin I, Bump RC. Validation of two global impression questionnaires for incontinence. Am J Obstet Gynecol. 2003;189(1):98–101.
48. Srikrishna S, Robinson D, Cardozo L. Validation of the patient global impression of improvement (PGI-I) for urogenital prolapse. Int Urogynecol J. 2010;21(5):523–8.
49. Trutnovsky G, et al. The "bother" of urinary incontinence. Int Urogynecol J. 2014;25(7):947–51.
50. Hagen S, et al. Psychometric properties of the pelvic organ prolapse symptom score. BJOG. 2009;116(1):25–31.

51. Hagen S, et al. Individualised pelvic floor muscle training in women with pelvic organ pro-
    lapse (POPPY): a multicentre randomised controlled trial. Lancet. 2014;383(9919):796–806.
52. Maher C. ICI 2012: pelvic organ prolapse surgery. Int Urogynecol J. 2013;24(11):1781.
53. Swift S, et al. Pelvic Organ Support Study (POSST): the distribution, clinical defini-
    tion, and epidemiologic condition of pelvic organ support defects. Am J Obstet Gynecol.
    2005;192(3):795–806.
54. Samuelsson EC, et al. Signs of genital prolapse in a Swedish population of women 20 to 59
    years of age and possible related factors. Am J Obstet Gynecol. 1999;180(2 Pt 1):299–305.
55. Culligan PJ, et al. A randomized controlled trial comparing fascia lata and synthetic mesh for
    sacral colpopexy. Obstet Gynecol. 2005;106(1):29–37.
56. Zyczynski HM, et al. One-year clinical outcomes after prolapse surgery with nonanchored
    mesh and vaginal support device. Am J Obstet Gynecol. 2010;203(6):587.e1–8.
57. Chmielewski L, et al. Reanalysis of a randomized trial of 3 techniques of anterior colpor-
    rhaphy using clinically relevant definitions of success. Am J Obstet Gynecol. 2011;205(1):69.
    e1–8.
58. Sayer T, et al. Medium-term clinical outcomes following surgical repair for vaginal prolapse
    with tension-free mesh and vaginal support device. Int Urogynecol J. 2012;23(4):487–93.
59. Macer GA. Transabdominal repair of cystocele, a 20 year experience, compared with the tra-
    ditional vaginal approach. Am J Obstet Gynecol. 1978;131(2):203–7.
60. Stanton SL, et al. Clinical and urodynamic effects of anterior colporrhaphy and vaginal hys-
    terectomy for prolapse with and without incontinence. Br J Obstet Gynaecol. 1982;89(6):
    459–63.
61. Walter S, et al. Urodynamic evaluation after vaginal repair and colposuspension. Br J Urol.
    1982;54(4):377–80.
62. Porges RF, Smilen SW. Long-term analysis of the surgical management of pelvic support
    defects. Am J Obstet Gynecol. 1994;171(6):1518–26; discussion 1526-8.
63. Sand PK, et al. Prospective randomized trial of polyglactin 910 mesh to prevent recurrence of
    cystoceles and rectoceles. Am J Obstet Gynecol. 2001;184(7):1357–62; discussion 1362-4.
64. Weber AM, et al. Anterior colporrhaphy: a randomized trial of three surgical techniques. Am J
    Obstet Gynecol. 2001;185(6):1299–304; discussion 1304-6.
65. Antosh DD, et al. Outcome assessment with blinded versus unblinded POP-Q exams. Am J
    Obstet Gynecol. 2011;205(5):489.e1–4.
66. Digesu GA, et al. The FIGO assessment scoring system (FASS): a new holistic classification
    tool to assess women with pelvic floor dysfunction: validity and reliability. Int Urogynecol J
    Pelvic Floor Dysfunct. 2015;26(6):859–64.
67. Olsen A, et al. Epidemiology of surgically managed pelvic organ prolapse and urinary incon-
    tinence. Obstet Gynecol. 1997;89(4):501–6.
68. Miedel A, et al. A 5-year prospective follow-up study of vaginal surgery for pelvic organ pro-
    lapse. Int Urogynecol J Pelvic Floor Dysfunct. 2008;19(12):1593–601.
69. Kapoor DS, et al. Reoperation rate for traditional anterior vaginal repair: analysis of 207 cases
    with a median 4-year follow-up. Int Urogynecol J. 2010;21(1):27–31.
70. Brubaker L, et al. Abdominal sacrocolpopexy with Burch colposuspension to reduce urinary
    stress incontinence. N Engl J Med. 2006;354(15):1557–66.
71. Maher C, et al. Surgical management of pelvic organ prolapse in women. Cochrane Database
    Syst Rev. 2004;4:CD004014.
72. Paraiso MF, et al. Pelvic support defects and visceral and sexual function in women treated
    with sacrospinous ligament suspension and pelvic reconstruction. Am J Obstet Gynecol.
    1996;175(6):1423–30; discussion 1430-1.
73. Barber MD, et al. Bilateral uterosacral ligament vaginal vault suspension with site-specific
    endopelvic fascia defect repair for treatment of pelvic organ prolapse. Am J Obstet Gynecol.
    2000;183(6):1402–10; discussion 1410-1.
74. U.S. Department of Health and Human Services FDA Center for Drug Evaluation and
    Research; U.S. Department of Health and Human Services FDA Center for Biologics
    Evaluation and Research; U.S. Department of Health and Human Services FDA Center for

Devices and Radiological Health. Guidance for industry patient-reported outcome measures: use in medical product development to support labeling claims: draft guidance. Health Qual Life Outcomes. 2006;4:79. SRC—GoogleScholar.

75. Doaee M, et al. Management of pelvic organ prolapse and quality of life: a systematic review and meta-analysis. Int Urogynecol J. 2014;25(2):153–63.

76. Altman D, et al. Sexual dysfunction after trocar-guided transvaginal mesh repair of pelvic organ prolapse. Obstet Gynecol. 2009;113(1):127–33.

77. Gauruder-Burmester A, et al. Follow-up after polypropylene mesh repair of anterior and posterior compartments in patients with recurrent prolapse. Int Urogynecol J Pelvic Floor Dysfunct. 2007;18(9):1059–64.

Urinary, Bowel and Sexual Symptoms After Surgery for Pelvic Organ Prolapse

14

Sharif I. M. F. Ismail and Diaa E. E. Rizk

14.1 Introduction

Urinary, bowel and sexual symptoms are important subjective outcome measures used to evaluate surgery for pelvic organ prolapse [POP] [1]. Establishing the effect of POP surgery on these symptoms can assist patients in judging the value of surgical management and help physicians in recommending the best surgical option for individual patients to meet their goals and expectations. Patients with POP may suffer from preoperative urinary, bowel and sexual symptoms, and surgical management of POP may be followed by improvement, worsening or no change in these symptoms. Alternatively, some patients with POP who do not have urinary, bowel or sexual problems may develop de novo symptoms postoperatively. This chapter will review the available evidence on the reported outcomes of surgical management of POP in relation to urinary, bowel and sexual symptoms in order to guide clinicians during preoperative counselling of women with POP.

14.2 Urinary Symptoms

A recent Cochrane systematic review concluded that there is no statistically significant increase in the probability of stress urinary incontinence [SUI] following anterior repair using native tissue (fascial) and biological mesh (RR 1.44, 95% CI 0.79–2.64), polypropylene mesh (RR 0.67, 95% CI 0.44–1.01) or absorbable mesh

S. I. M. F. Ismail, MSc, MD, FRCOG (✉)
Brighton and Sussex University Hospitals NHS Trust, Brighton and Sussex Medical School, Brighton, UK

D. E. E. Rizk, MSc, FRCOG, FRCS, MD
Department of Obstetrics and Gynaecology, College of Medicine and Medical sciences, Arabian Gulf University, Manama, Kingdom of Bahrain

© Springer International Publishing AG, part of Springer Nature 2018
V. Li Marzi, M. Serati (eds.), *Management of Pelvic Organ Prolapse*,
Urodynamics, Neurourology and Pelvic Floor Dysfunctions,
https://doi.org/10.1007/978-3-319-59195-7_14

(RR 0.72, 95% CI 0.50–1.05) [2]. A previous systematic review by the same group had also shown that anterior fascial repair is followed by less de novo SUI than armed mesh repair [3]. As regards apical prolapse, SUI was more common after vaginal surgery compared to abdominal or laparoscopic surgery (RR 1.86, 95% CI 1.17–2.94) [4]. There was no statistically significant difference, however, in the need for SUI surgery after vaginal mesh repair compared to native tissue repair of apical prolapse (RR 4.91, 95% CI 0.86–27.94).

There was no significant difference in the postoperative outcome between combined and interval surgery for POP and SUI in women with POP and coexistent (symptomatic) SUI [5]. For women with occult SUI, combined surgery was followed with a significantly lower incidence of de novo subjective SUI (RR 0.6, 95% CI 0.3–0.9) and need for subsequent anti-incontinence surgery (RR 0.4, 95% CI 0.2–0.8) but without a statistically significant difference in objective SUI rates, overactive bladder symptoms [OAB] or voiding dysfunction. However, a statistically significant increase in adverse events (RR 1.6, 95% CI 1.0–2.5) and prolonged catheterisation (RR 4.5, 95% CI 1.5–13.3) were observed in these women after combined POP and SUI surgery.

Preoperative OAB symptoms may resolve in 40% of patients following POP repair. However, de novo OAB symptoms and voiding dysfunction may develop in 12% [3] and 9% of these patients, respectively [6].

14.3 Bowel Symptoms

A prospective study involving 65 women who had a variety of surgical procedures for POP repair including anterior repair (36), posterior repair (32), sacrocolpopexy (13) and vaginal hysterectomy (20) showed significant improvement in bowel symptoms such as constipation, straining and digitations at 30 months follow-up [7]. Another prospective study of the effect of posterior repair on bowel symptoms in 60 women evaluated by the electronic Personal Assessment Questionnaire-Pelvic Floor (ePAQ-PF) found a significant improvement in bowel evacuation (42%), continence (37%) and bowel-related quality of life (61%) scores at 3–6 months follow-up [8]. Although irritable bowel scores improved by 28% in these women, this was not statistically significant. There was also no significant change in constipation (0.5%). All other bowel evacuation and continence symptoms, however, improved significantly except for painful evacuation and incontinence to solid stool. A recent systematic review and meta-analysis found no statistically significant difference in bowel symptoms, however, after mesh sacrocolpopexy or fascial pelvic floor repair at 6 months follow-up [9].

In the extended Colpopexy And urinary Reduction Effort (e-CARE) trial, there was significant improvement in obstructed defecation 5 years after abdominal sacrocolpopexy regardless of whether a posterior repair was carried out at surgery or not, despite that obstructed defecation was present in up to 17%–19% of patients at follow-up [10]. Another retrospective cohort study of 238 women who underwent anterior/apical prolapse surgery of whom 61 (26%) underwent a concomitant posterior repair showed significant improvement of the Colorectal-Anal Distress Inventory (CRADI-8) scores at 6 weeks postoperatively [11]. A significantly larger margin of symptom improvement was noted in those who underwent posterior repair as compared to those who did not (18.2 ± 20.1 vs. 9.9 ± 18.6, $P < 0.01$). On linear regression modelling, these women scored 4.9 points lower on the postoperative CRADI-8 score which suggests better improvement in bowel-related symptoms (95% confidence interval, 1.0–8.8, $P = 0.02$). Resolution of preoperative outlet constipation was observed n 56% of patients in a cohort study of 77 women having robotic sacrocolpopexy with or without concomitant posterior repair without a statistically significant difference between both groups [12]. The rate of postoperative de novo outlet constipation was, however, relatively high: 13.6%.

A prospective study looked at the effect of colpocleisis on bowel function at 1-year follow-up using the Colorectal-Anal Distress Inventory (CRADI) and the Colorectal-Anal Impact Questionnaire (CRAIQ) [13]. The study included 121 patients, 74 (61%) had partial colpocleisis and 47 (39%) had total colpocleisis with additional levator myorrhaphy in 86 (71%) and perineorrhaphy in 117 (97%). All bothersome obstructive and anal incontinence symptoms were less prevalent 1 year after surgery. The rate of faecal urgency, passage of mucus with bowel movements and haemorrhoids was also significantly reduced. However, no statistically significant difference was noted in pain prior to bowel movement or with defecation and straining. CRADI and CRAIQ scores significantly improved, and the rate of de novo symptoms was low (0–14%).

14.4   Sexual Symptoms

It is important to establish the baseline sexual function accurately before POP surgery, preferably using validated condition specific questionnaires [14], counsel patients properly to appreciate their problems and guide their expectations [15]. The potential for husband/partner dyspareunia (hispareunia) with mesh complications, such as mesh exposure, also needs to be taken into consideration [16].

A systematic review and meta-analysis showed significant improvement in sexual function following fascial repair for POP (standardised mean difference −0.55, 95% CI −0.68 to −0.43), with improvement in the rate of dyspareunia (OR > 2.5) [17]. Overall, 47% of women had improvement, 39% no change, 18% deterioration and 4% new-onset dyspareunia postoperatively. The chance of improvement or no change was 4.8 times higher than that of deterioration.

In another Cochrane systematic review, a significantly higher incidence of dyspareunia was observed after vaginal than abdominal or laparoscopic repair of apical compartment prolapse (RR 2.53, 95% CI 1.17–5.50) [4]. There was no significant difference, however, between the incidence of dyspareunia following mesh and non-mesh vaginal surgery for apical compartment prolapse [4]. Furthermore, the incidence of dyspareunia did no significantly increase following fascial and biological mesh anterior repair (RR 0.87, 95% CI 0.39–1.93) or polypropylene mesh anterior repair (RR 0.54, 95% CI 0.27–1.06) with no data available in relation to absorbable mesh anterior repair. A randomised controlled study showed no statistically significant difference in Pelvic Organ Prolapse/Urinary Incontinence Sexual Questionnaire (PISQ-12) scores at 1 and 3 years follow-up after fascial repair and collagen-coated prolene mesh repair as primary procedures for anterior compartment prolapse [18]. Although significantly more women were sexually active in the fascial repair group compare to the mesh group (37.3% vs. 32.3%, $P < 0.01$) at 3 years follow-up, there was no significant difference between both groups in decline of sexual activity at 1 year. A previous review supported these findings and concluded that the use of both absorbable and non-absorbable meshes for anterior repair has no significant detrimental effect on sexual function in comparison to fascial repair [19]. As regards posterior compartment prolapse, a literature review concluded that there are insufficient studies to provide evidence-based conclusions on the effect of mesh repair on sexual symptoms [19].

In a registry-based study of 726 transvaginal mesh procedures for POP with ten different kits between 2006 and 2010, dyspareunia was reported by 7 and 10% of 265 and 181 sexually active patients, respectively, at 3 and 12 months postoperatively [20]. In a retrospective review of 398 procedures performed for the removal of vaginal mesh at a single tertiary centre over 75 months between January 2008 and April 2014, dyspareunia was the primary indication in 57% of cases [21]. Dyspareunia was also noted in 82.2% of sexually active women presenting with mesh complications in another retrospective study of 79 women evaluated by endovaginal ultrasound [22]. Mesh removal was followed by resolution of dyspareunia in 3 out of 23 (13%) sexually active women in another study [23].

Conclusion

Assessment of urinary, bowel and sexual symptoms is an integral component of both preoperative counselling and postoperative evaluation of patients with pelvic organ prolapse.

Prolapse repair using native tissue or mesh does not appear to increase the risk of de novo postoperative stress urinary incontinence with the highest probability occurring after vaginal repair of apical prolapse. Women with prolapse and coexistent symptomatic stress urinary incontinence should be informed that there is no difference in the postoperative outcome of combined and interval anti-incontinence surgery and the treatment plan individualized. Patients with occult stress urinary incontinence should be counselled that combined surgery is followed by a lower incidence of incontinence at the expense of greater postoperative adverse events in order to choose the best treatment option. Preoperative overactive bladder symptoms and voiding dysfunction usually resolve after prolapse repair although a minority of patients may develop these de novo manifestations postoperatively.

Prolapse surgery, whether pelvic floor repair or colpocleisis, is associated with significant improvement in bowel symptoms, at least in the short term. The effect is greater if a concomitant posterior repair is performed but with a higher risk of postoperative de novo constipation.

The evidence on sexual function after prolapse surgery is less clear with conflicting results reported in the literature, but the effect seems to depend on the affected compartment. Sexual symptoms, particularly dyspareunia, tends to improve after abdominal or laparoscopic repair of apical compartment prolapse. The effect of transvaginal mesh repair, as opposed to native tissue repair, on sexual function is controversial, and the data available are mainly related to anterior compartment prolapse. Some reports showed no significant detrimental effect of anterior compartment mesh repair, whilst others described high postoperative dyspareunia and mesh removal request rates. The studies on the effect of posterior compartment repair on sexual function are limited, which precludes making evidence-based recommendations. Until more robust data are available on the effect of prolapse surgery on sexual function, careful preoperative counselling with a patient-centred approach for treatment decisions is advisable.

References

1. Barber MD, Brubaker L, Nygaard I, Wheeler TL 2nd, Schaffer J, Chen Z, Spino C, Pelvic Floor Disorders Network. Defining success after surgery for pelvic organ prolapse. Obstet Gynecol. 2009;114:600–9.
2. Maher C, Feiner B, Baessler K, Christmann-Schmid C, Haya N, Brown J. Surgery for women with anterior compartment prolapse. Cochrane Database Syst Rev. 2016;11:CD004014.
3. Baessler K, Maher C. Pelvic organ prolapse surgery and bladder function. Int Urogynecol J. 2013;24:1843–52.
4. Maher C, Feiner B, Baessler K, Christmann-Schmid C, Haya N, Brown J. Surgery for women with apical vaginal prolapse. Cochrane Database Syst Rev. 2016a;10:CD012376.
5. van der Ploeg JM, van der Steen A, Oude Rengerink K, van der Vaart CH, Roovers JP. Prolapse surgery with or without stress incontinence surgery for pelvic organ prolapse: a systematic review and meta-analysis of randomised trials. BJOG. 2014;121:537–47.
6. Maher C, Feiner B, Baessler K, Schmid C. Surgical management of pelvic organ prolapse in women. Cochrane Database Syst Rev. 2013;4:CD004014.
7. de Oliveira MS, Cavalcanti Gde A, da Costa AA. Native vaginal tissue repair for genital prolapse surgical treatment: a minimum of 30 months of results. Eur J Obstet Gynecol Reprod Biol. 2016;201:75–8.
8. Dua A, Radley S, Brown S, Jha S, Jones G. The effect of posterior colporrhaphy on anorectal function. Int Urogynecol J. 2012;23:749–53.
9. Siddiqui NY, Grimes CL, Casiano ER, Abed HT, Jeppson PC, Olivera CK, Sanses TV, Steinberg AC, South MM, Balk EM, Sung VW, Society of Gynecologic Surgeons Systematic Review Group. Mesh sacrocolpopexy compared with native tissue vaginal repair: a systematic review and meta-analysis. Obstet Gynecol. 2015;125:44–55.
10. Grimes CL, Lukacz ES, Gantz MG, Warren LK, Brubaker L, Zyczynski HM, Richter HE, Jelovsek JE, Cundiff G, Fine P, Visco AG, Zhang M, Meikle S, NICHD Pelvic Floor Disorders Network. What happens to the posterior compartment and bowel symptoms after sacrocolpopexy? evaluation of 5-year outcomes from E-CARE. Female Pelvic Med Reconstr Surg. 2014;20:261–6.
11. Edenfield AL, Levin PJ, Dieter AA, Wu JM, Siddiqui NY. Is postoperative bowel function related to posterior compartment prolapse repair? Female Pelvic Med Reconstr Surg. 2014;20:90–4.
12. Crane AK, Geller EJ, Matthews CA. Outlet constipation 1 year after robotic sacrocolpopexy with and without concomitant posterior repair. South Med J. 2013;106:409–14.
13. Gutman RE, Bradley CS, Ye W, Markland AD, Whitehead WE, Fitzgerald MP, Network PFD. Effects of colpocleisis on bowel symptoms among women with severe pelvic organ prolapse. Int Urogynecol J. 2010;21:461–6.

14. Kammerer-Doak D. Assessment of sexual function in women with pelvic floor dysfunction. Int Urogynecol J. 2009;20(Suppl 1):S45–50.
15. Karmakar D, Dwyer PL. Failure of expectations in vaginal surgery: lack of appropriate consent, goals and expectations of surgery. Curr Urol Rep. 2016;17:87.
16. Petri E, Ashok K. Partner dyspareunia: a report of six cases. Int Urogynecol J. 2012;23:127–9.
17. Jha S, Gray T. A systematic review and meta-analysis of the impact of native tissue repair for pelvic organ prolapse on sexual function. Int Urogynecol J. 2015;26:321–7.
18. Rudnicki M, Laurikainen E, Pogosean R, Kinne I, Jakobsson U, Teleman P. A 3-year follow-up after anterior colporrhaphy compared with collagen-coated transvaginal mesh for anterior vaginal wall prolapse: a randomised controlled trial. BJOG. 2016;123:136–42.
19. Dietz V, Maher C. Pelvic organ prolapse and sexual function. Int Urogynecol J. 2013;24: 1853–7.
20. Bjelic-Radisic V, Aigmueller T, Preyer O, Ralph G, Geiss I, Muller G, Riss P, Klug P, Konrad M, Wagner G, Medl M, Umek W, Lozano P, Tamussino K, Tammaa A, Austrian Urogynecology Working Group. Vaginal prolapse surgery with transvaginal mesh: results of the Austrian registry. Int Urogynecol J. 2014;25:1047–52.
21. Pickett SD, Barenberg B, Quiroz LH, Shobeiri SA, O'Leary DE. The significant morbidity of removing pelvic mesh from multiple vaginal compartments. Obstet Gynecol. 2015;125:1418–22.
22. Manonai J, Rostaminia G, Denson L, Shobeiri SA. Clinical and ultrasonographic study of patients presenting with transvaginal mesh complications. Neurourol Urodyn. 2016;35:407–11.
23. Hokenstad ED, El-Nashar SA, Blandon RE, Occhino JA, Trabuco EC, Gebhart JB, Klingele CJ. Health-related quality of life and outcomes after surgical treatment of complications from vaginally placed mesh. Female Pelvic Med Reconstr Surg. 2015;21:176–80.

Index

© Springer International Publishing AG, part of Springer Nature 2018   173
V. Li Marzi, M. Serati (eds.), *Management of Pelvic Organ Prolapse*,
Urodynamics, Neurourology and Pelvic Floor Dysfunctions,
https://doi.org/10.1007/978-3-319-59195-7

The manufacturer's authorised representative in the EU is Springer
Nature Customer Service Centre GmbH, Europaplatz 3, 69115 Heidelberg,
Germany. If you have any concerns regarding our products, please
contact ProductSafety@springernature.com

Printed and bound by CPI Group (UK) Ltd, Croydon, CR0 4YY
29/04/2026
02099516-0001